TAP *IT* OUT

Taking Baby-Steps to Better

Self-Care and Empowerment
Guided EFT

6x9 Journal

ISBN: 9798640278385
Independently published

DEDICATION

To you, your family, and all of us in the human family.
May we find more peace and true joy today.
One baby step at a time

Why are you tapping?
Who are you dedicating your tapping work to?

CONTENTS

HOW TO EFT

Websites/Pdf's of How to do EFT/Tapping:

There are so many resources for learning EFT. If you google "EFT TAPPING PDF" you'll find many resources that'll teach you how to do this. Also, the books you can find online, on Amazon, Thriftbooks, Abebooks, etc. are more than enough to help you succeed.

Here are free online resources that were available at the time of printing this book:

- www.thetappingsolution.com/TappingSolutionEbook.pdf

- https://eftinternational.org/wp-content/uploads/EFT-International-Free-Tapping-Manual.pdf

- http://www.lifecoachingwithlindsay.com/downloads/Level1_Workbook_FINAL.pdf

- http://www.eft-alive.com/how-to-do-EFT.html

- https://grapevinecenter.org/alternative-views-resources/eft/

RESOURCING

Resourcing and Self-Care, are an important part of healing, optimized living where you consciously choose actions that help you thrive.

For this exercise "RESOURCING" means you identify and use your internal and external resources —things that delight or relax you, things that help you feel centered and balanced, energized, happy and capable.

Write down what your Resources are, then use some or one of them on a daily basis. Doing this strengthens your brain's natural ability to process life in a healthy way

Here are some ideas to get you started as you write or add to your personal list of things that delight you, balance you, calm or sooth you, enliven you, activities or thoughts that help you feel and be productive, alive and connected.

Internal Resources Ideas	External Resources Ideas	
Detailed Positive Memories of being with someone safe, fun, happy, energizing	Gardening	Reading'
	Singing	Weight
	Games	Lifting
	Playing Music	Knitting
Image of a Safe Place, imagining you there	Walking	Sewing
	Dancing	Crafting'
	Massage	Drawing
Spiritual Guide Connection, connection to God	Essential Oils	Painting
	Yawn and Stretch	Live Theater
	Friend time	Writing
Other places you can go to in your mind and heart	Take a Class	Meditating
	Sports	Pet time
	Yoga	Swing
	Hiking	
	Nature walks	
	Forest Bathing	
	Dog Walking	
	Cooking	
	Bubble Bath	
	Epsom Salt Bath	
	Mantra	
	Doodling	
	Horseback Riding	
	Nap	

Internal Resources	External Resources

6

~ Baby Steps to Better ~

EMOTIONS

Name the emotion your issue brings up

GUILTY	DISGUSTED	DISTRUSTFUL
Accountable	abhorred.	Apprehension
Apologetic	appalled.	Astonished
At fault	Aversion	Confusion
Avoiding	Detestable	Disbelief
Bad	Disapproving	Disillusioned
Blamed	Disgraceful	Distrust
Caught	displeased.	doubt
Convicted	Grossed out	Fear
Corrupt	Hateful	Hesitant
Liable	Loathsome	Judgmental
Meek	outraged.	Loathing
Mischievous	queasy.	Perplexed
Naughty	Rejecting	Provocative
offensive	Revolted	Reluctance
Remorseful	scandalous	Repugnant
responsible	tired.	Sarcastic
Shameful	unhappy.	Skeptical
Wrong	Vile	Suspicious
	weary	uncertain
		Wary

VULNERABLE/HURT		MAD/ANGER
Annoyed	Resentful	aggressive
Avoiding	Sensitive	angry
Awful	Submissive	berated
Broken	Susceptible	covetous
Confused	Threatened	critical
Constricted	Tight	cruel
Damaged	Unhappy	disappointed
Defenseless	Unprotected	disapproving
Dejected	Unsafe	distant
Disturbed	weak	enraged
down	Withdrawn	frustrated
Exposed	Wronged	furious
Fragile		hateful
Grieved		hostile
Helpless		hurt
Hidden		infuriated
Humiliated		irate
Hurt		irritated
Ignored		jealous
Indifferent		mad
Insecure		pissed
Irritated		provoked
Offended		resentful
Pained		sarcastic
Powerless		selfish
Raw		skeptical
Rejected		violated

SCARED/AFRAID	SAD	ASHAMED
Afraid	Abandoned	Alienated
Anxious	Alone	Devastated
Anxious	Apathetic	Disrespected
Bewildered	Ashamed	Distressed
Confused	Bored	Embarrassed
Discouraged	Depressed	Empty
Dismayed	Despairing	Guilty
Embarrassed	Disappointed	Humiliated
Fearful	Droopy	Inadequate
Frightened	Empty	Inferior
Helpless	Flat	Insecure
Hesitant	Guilty	Insignificant
Inadequate	Ignored	Isolated
Insecure	Inferior	Mortified
Insignificant	Isolated	Powerless
Overwhelmed	Lonely	Regret
Rejected	remorseful	Remorseful
Shocked	Sleepy	Ridiculed
Startled	Stupid	Shamefaced
Submissive	Tired	Sheepish
Terrified	Withdrawn	Sorry
worried		Uncomfortable
		Victimized
		Withdrawn
		Worthless

12

SENSATIONS

Label the pain or sensation associated with the
issue/memory/problem
Note the location, size, shape and the edges of the pain.
Where does it NOT hurt?

Here are lists of sensations that may help you identify what you feel:

ANXIETY	VULNERABLE/HURT	TENDER
Clammy	Achy	Aglow
Dizzy	Brittle	Bruised
Flushed	Bruised	Cozy
Fluttery	Cutting	Melting
Frantic	Open	Moved
Nauseous	Piercing	Tender
Nervous	Prickly	Touched
Paralyzed	Raw	Warm
Pit in stomach	Searing	
Queasy	Sensitive	
Quivery	Sore	
Spacey	Trembly	
Tingling	Wobbly	
Twitchy		

ANGRY	CONSTRICTED	
Burning	Achy	Pinching
Churning	Armored	Pounding
Clenched	Blocked	Pressing
Constricted	Clenched	Pressure
Dense	Closed	Restricted
Energized	Cold	Stiff
Explosive	Congested	Stuck
Fiery	Constricted	Suffocated
Gnawing	Contracted	Tense
Hot	Cool	Thick
Impulsive	Cramped	Throbbing
Knotted	Jammed	Tight
Red hot	Knotted	Wooden
Rush	Numb	
Stuck		
Twisted		
Wrenching		

SCARED	SAD	SHAME/DEPRESSED
Breathless	Alone	Alone
Cold	Blue	Contracted
Dark	Burdened	Crushing
Faint	Closed	Cut-off
Frozen	Empty	Deflated
Jittery	Heavy	Disappearing
Jumpy	Hole	Disconnected
Shaky	Hollow	Draining
Shivery	Piercing	Dull
Sweaty	Untethered	Empty
Trembling	Weighted	Fragile
		Frozen
		Heavy
		Hiding
		Hollow
		Icy
		Imploding
		Numb
		Small
		Worn out

ENERGIZED		OPENHEARTED
Activate	Radiating	Airy
Breathless	Referring	Alive
Bubbly	Releasing	Awake
Buzzy	Shaky	Bubbly
Electric	Shimmery	Calm
Energized	Tearing	Expanded
Floating	Throbbing	Expansive
Fluid	Tingling	Flowing
Heated	Tingling	Fluid
Itchy	Tingly	Full
Luminous	Tremulous	Light
Nervy	Twitchy	Open
Pounding	Warm	Relaxed
Prickly		Relaxed
Pulsing		Releasing
		Shimmering
		Smooth
		Spacious
		Still
		Vital

MISC.		
Bloated	Jagged	Spacious
Cool		Spinning
Damp	Light	Still
Dark	Moist	Streaming
Deep	Penetrating	Stringy
Dense	Puffy	Strong
Dry	Pulling	Sweaty
Flaccid	Radiating	Thick
Floating	Ragged	Thin
Full	Referring	Squeezing
Fuzzy	Sharp	Stabbing
Hot	Shooting	Stinging
Icy	Smooth	Tugging
Inflated	Sore	
	Spacey	

18

PERSONALIZED TAPPING LISTS

What it IT that hangs you up? That disrupts relationships, slows down your life, leaves you feeling 'less than'? What is IT? It's time to list all those IT's AND all the excuses not to release them!

This becomes your master Tapping List. Tapping on one or two a day (*Baby Steps*, remember?) will bring you greater peace, allow your body to process the work you're doing, and, months from now, leave you wondering what those IT's were that had you so stuck and feeling crummy.

You could start with these first two lists, then move on to your own master list.

Common Blocks to EFT Success (tap on these as needed)

- I don't believe these treatments will work.
- I believe EFT works, but not for me.
- I doubt that EFT will work.
- Even if EFT does work, I am afraid it won't last.
- I don't trust myself to stay free of these problems now.
- I am afraid that these treatments won't work.
- I am afraid that the problem will come back.
- I'm afraid to give up my hopelessness, helplessness, fear, etc.
- I doubt it will happen.
- I'm supposed to be rejected.
- I don't trust myself to live it out.
- I'm supposed to be disapproved of.
- I don't feel safe with ... (whatever the situation is)
- I have to be perfect about everything.
- I fear something like this problem will happen again.
- I doubt that I will really be able to do this.

Limiting Beliefs
Limiting Beliefs add another element to address.
There are a few steps to be aware of:

Common Limiting Beliefs

- I can't because...
- I don't deserve...
- I don't have enough...
- I don't have time
- I have to play small
- I must be in control
- I'll never measure up
- I'm a burden
- I'm a failure
- I'm a procrastinator
- I'm a quitter.
- I'm a sinner
- I'm a victim
- I'm abandoned
- I'm alone
- I'm always broke
- I'm always used
- I'm bad
- I'm betrayed
- I'm broken
- I'm confused
- I'm defective
- I'm dumb
- I'm guilty
- I'm incapable
- I'm incompetent
- I'm inferior
- I'm just not motivated
- I'm lazy
- I'm misunderstood
- I'm not good enough
- I'm not loveable
- I'm not...
- I'm poor
- I'm powerless
- I'm separated from God
- I'm stupid
- I'm too...
- I'm trapped
- I'm ugly
- I'm unattractive
- I'm unproductive
- I'm worthless
- If I succeed, I won't be able to sustain it
- Love hurts
- My body betrayed me
- Nobody cares what I have to say
- Now is not the time.
- People will judge me
- The world is dangerous

Not Making Progress?
Address Psychological Reversals:
(tap on these as needed)

- Do I keep the problem to get sympathy that I won't get if I release the problem?
- Does keeping the problem allow me to avoid unpleasant situations or responsibilities?
- Does keeping the problem give me financial rewards that I won't receive without it?
- Do I feel I don't deserve to get over the problem?
- Do I fear that if I get better, something bad will happen?
- Can I give myself permission to get over this problem?
- Who will be upset if I get over this problem?
- Do I care if they get upset, or am I pandering to them?
- How will getting over this problem change my life?
- What benefits do you receive from your problem?
- Does keeping the problem feel safe?
- Does releasing it feel dangerous?
- Am I afraid to let it go?
- Do I want these changes?
- Do I believe that I will be able to keep these changes?

SELF ACCEPTANCE PHRASES

"Even though ___,I deeply and completely) accept myself"
is the standard acceptance phrase to use, but not every situation or person resonates with that.
Trust yourself and use one that works for you and your situation.

EVEN THOUGH...,

- I know EFT will shift this as it has so many times before
- I want to (deeply and completely) accept myself (anyway)
- I (deeply and) completely love and accept myself.
- I can accept that this is just where I am right now
- I accept that I feel this way
- I want to love and accept myself with compassion
- I can choose to be a little kinder to myself
- I accept all my feelings without judgment
- I can love and accept all parts of me
- I love and accept my young self
- I'm ok anyway (I'll be OK).
- I'll feel better soon.
- everything's improving
- it's time to bring some healing to this
- this is where I am at right now
- I can let these feelings safely flow
- I'm open to the possibility of ________
- I'm willing for this to transform
- I   someday be willing to entertain the slight possibility of__
- I honor myself for how hard it has been

TAPPING SESSIONS

The Prompts in the journal will help identify these areas so that you don't have to pause and think about them when you are tapping:

1. Give the event/Condition/Problem a 'Movie' Title

2. Identify the Emotions in response

3. Identify the Origin, Location and Source of Emotion in the body

4. Self- Acceptance statement ("Even though…,)

Date___________

THE PROBLEM's "MOVIE TITLE"

THE NEGATIVE BELIEF/SELF-TALK:

Rate it: 1-100 (1= least intense, 100 = most intense)

CONSIDER THE DETAILS (past/present/future):

WHAT event/condition happened?	WHEN did it start?
WHO was/will be involved?	WHAT was/is going on?
WHERE did/will it happen?	WHY did/will it happen?
WHEN did/will it happen?	HOW did/will it happen?

What does this REMIND me of?	What OTHER ISSUES came up?
What is the EARLIEST MEMORY this reminds me of?	What other SELF TALK attends this?

What EMOTION & BODY SENSATIONS do I feel/notice?

Where is this felt?

Size? Shape? Edges?

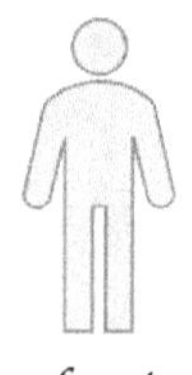 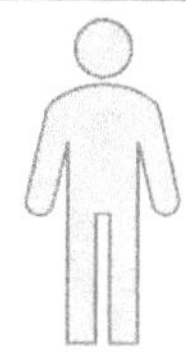

front   *back*

Intensity of Emotion BEFORE tapping:

1 2 3 4 5 6 7 8 9 10   Low – Medium – High

SET UP STATEMENT: 3x's at side of hand

"Even though

,*I deeply and completely accept myself"

Self-Acceptance Phrase

REMINDER PHRASE: at all other points

"This   in my

CHECK INTENSITY OF EMOTION: check after each round

Set Up for Additional Tapping as needed

"Even though *I have some remaining* __________, I deeply and completely accept myself."

"This *remaining* _______.

NOTES: ____

____

____

____

____

____

____

____

____

Date___________

THE PROBLEM's "MOVIE TITLE"

THE NEGATIVE BELIEF/SELF-TALK:

Rate it: 1-100 (1= least intense, 100 = most intense)

CONSIDER THE DETAILS (past/present/future):

WHAT event/condition happened?	WHEN did it start?
WHO was/will be involved?	WHAT was/is going on?
WHERE did/will it happen?	WHY did/will it happen?
WHEN did/will it happen?	HOW did/will it happen?

What does this REMIND me of?	What OTHER ISSUES came up?
What is the EARLIEST MEMORY this reminds me of?	What other SELF TALK attends this?

What EMOTION & BODY SENSATIONS do I feel/notice?

Where is this felt?

Size? Shape? Edges?

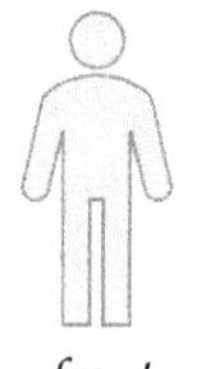
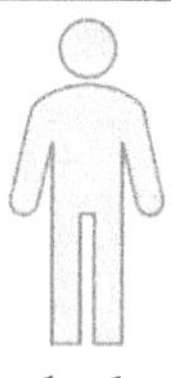

front   *back*

Intensity of Emotion BEFORE tapping:

1 2 3 4 5 6 7 8 9 10   Low – Medium – High

SET UP STATEMENT: 3x's at side of hand

"Even though

,*I deeply and completely accept myself"

Self-Acceptance Phrase

REMINDER PHRASE: at all other points

"This   in my

CHECK INTENSITY OF EMOTION: check after each round

Set Up for Additional Tapping as needed

"Even though ***I have some remaining*** _________, I deeply and completely accept myself."

"This ***remaining*** _______.

NOTES: ____

____

____

____

____

____

____

____

____

Date____________

<table>
<tr><td>

THE PROBLEM's "MOVIE TITLE"

</td></tr>
</table>

<table>
<tr><td>

THE NEGATIVE BELIEF/SELF-TALK:

</td></tr>
<tr><td>

Rate it: 1-100 (1= least intense, 100 = most intense)

</td></tr>
</table>

<table>
<tr><td colspan="2">

CONSIDER THE DETAILS (past/present/future):

</td></tr>
<tr><td>

WHAT event/condition happened?

WHO was/will be involved?

WHERE did/will it happen?

WHEN did/will it happen?

</td><td>

WHEN did it start?

WHAT was/is going on?

WHY did/will it happen?

HOW did/will it happen?

</td></tr>
<tr><td>

What does this REMIND me of?

What is the EARLIEST MEMORY this reminds me of?

</td><td>

What OTHER ISSUES came up?

What other SELF TALK attends this?

</td></tr>
</table>

<table>
<tr><td colspan="2">

What EMOTION & BODY SENSATIONS do I feel/notice?

</td></tr>
<tr><td>

Where is this felt?

Size? Shape? Edges?

</td><td>

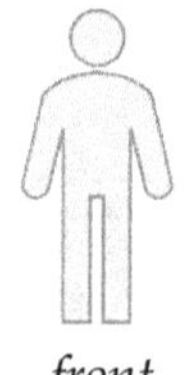 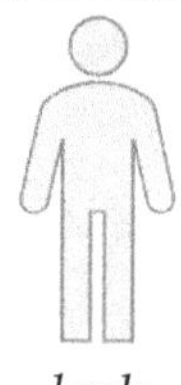

front   *back*

</td></tr>
<tr><td colspan="2">

Intensity of Emotion BEFORE tapping:

1 2 3 4 5 6 7 8 9 10   Low – Medium – High

</td></tr>
</table>

SET UP STATEMENT: 3x's at side of hand

"Even though

,*I deeply and completely accept myself"

Self-Acceptance Phrase

REMINDER PHRASE: at all other points

"This   in my

CHECK INTENSITY OF EMOTION: check after each round

Set Up for Additional Tapping as needed

"Even though **I have some remaining** _________, I deeply and completely accept myself."

"This **remaining** _______.

NOTES: ____

____

____

____

____

____

____

____

Date___________

THE PROBLEM's "MOVIE TITLE"

THE NEGATIVE BELIEF/SELF-TALK:

Rate it: 1-100 (1= least intense, 100 = most intense)

CONSIDER THE DETAILS (past/present/future):

WHAT event/condition happened?	WHEN did it start?
WHO was/will be involved?	WHAT was/is going on?
WHERE did/will it happen?	WHY did/will it happen?
WHEN did/will it happen?	HOW did/will it happen?

What does this REMIND me of?	What OTHER ISSUES came up?
What is the EARLIEST MEMORY this reminds me of?	What other SELF TALK attends this?

What EMOTION & BODY SENSATIONS do I feel/notice?

Where is this felt?

Size? Shape? Edges?

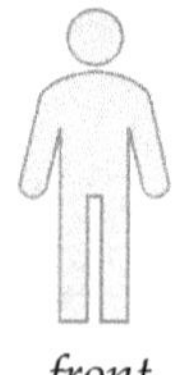 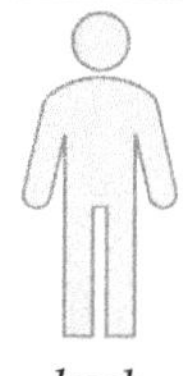

front   *back*

Intensity of Emotion BEFORE tapping:

1 2 3 4 5 6 7 8 9 10   Low – Medium – High

SET UP STATEMENT: 3x's at side of hand

"Even though

,*I deeply and completely accept myself"

Self-Acceptance Phrase

REMINDER PHRASE: at all other points

"This   in my

CHECK INTENSITY OF EMOTION: check after each round

Set Up for Additional Tapping as needed

"Even though ***I have some remaining*** _________, I deeply and completely accept myself."

"This ***remaining*** _______.

NOTES: _______________________________________

____

____

____

____

____

____

____

____

Date___________

<table>
<tr><td>

THE PROBLEM's "MOVIE TITLE"

</td></tr>
</table>

<table>
<tr><td>

THE NEGATIVE BELIEF/SELF-TALK:

Rate it: 1-100 (1= least intense, 100 = most intense)

</td></tr>
</table>

CONSIDER THE DETAILS (past/present/future):

WHAT event/condition happened?	WHEN did it start?
WHO was/will be involved?	WHAT was/is going on?
WHERE did/will it happen?	WHY did/will it happen?
WHEN did/will it happen?	HOW did/will it happen?

What does this REMIND me of?	What OTHER ISSUES came up?
What is the EARLIEST MEMORY this reminds me of?	What other SELF TALK attends this?

What EMOTION & BODY SENSATIONS do I feel/notice?

Where is this felt?

Size? Shape? Edges?

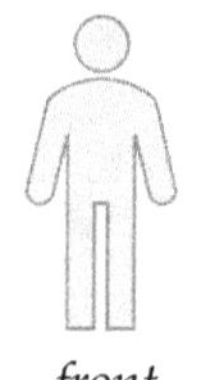
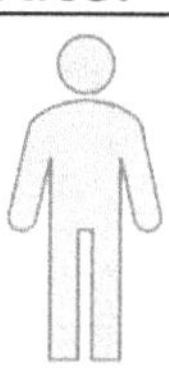

front   *back*

Intensity of Emotion BEFORE tapping:

1 2 3 4 5 6 7 8 9 10   Low – Medium – High

SET UP STATEMENT: 3x's at side of hand

"Even though

,*I deeply and completely accept myself"

Self-Acceptance Phrase

REMINDER PHRASE: at all other points

"This   in my

CHECK INTENSITY OF EMOTION: check after each round

Set Up for Additional Tapping as needed

"Even though **I have some remaining** _________, I deeply and completely accept myself."

"This **remaining** ______.

NOTES: _______________________________________

____

____

____

____

____

____

____

____

Date___________

THE PROBLEM's "MOVIE TITLE"

THE NEGATIVE BELIEF/SELF-TALK:

Rate it: 1-100 (1= least intense, 100 = most intense)

CONSIDER THE DETAILS (past/present/future):

WHAT event/condition happened?	WHEN did it start?
WHO was/will be involved?	WHAT was/is going on?
WHERE did/will it happen?	WHY did/will it happen?
WHEN did/will it happen?	HOW did/will it happen?

What does this REMIND me of?	What OTHER ISSUES came up?
What is the EARLIEST MEMORY this reminds me of?	What other SELF TALK attends this?

What EMOTION & BODY SENSATIONS do I feel/notice?

Where is this felt?

Size? Shape? Edges?

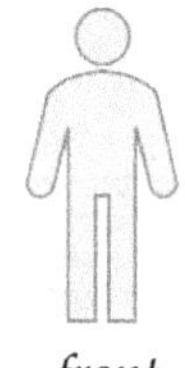 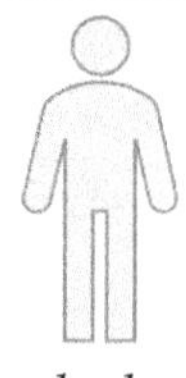

front   *back*

Intensity of Emotion BEFORE tapping:

1 2 3 4 5 6 7 8 9 10   Low – Medium – High

SET UP STATEMENT: 3x's at side of hand

"Even though

,*I deeply and completely accept myself"

Self-Acceptance Phrase

REMINDER PHRASE: at all other points

"This   in my

CHECK INTENSITY OF EMOTION: check after each round

Set Up for Additional Tapping as needed

"Even though **I have some remaining** __________, I deeply and completely accept myself."

"This **remaining** ______.

NOTES: ____

____

____

____

____

____

____

____

____

Date______________

THE PROBLEM's "MOVIE TITLE"

THE NEGATIVE BELIEF/SELF-TALK:

Rate it: 1-100 (1= least intense, 100 = most intense)

CONSIDER THE DETAILS (past/present/future):

WHAT event/condition happened?	WHEN did it start?
WHO was/will be involved?	WHAT was/is going on?
WHERE did/will it happen?	WHY did/will it happen?
WHEN did/will it happen?	HOW did/will it happen?

What does this REMIND me of?	What OTHER ISSUES came up?
What is the EARLIEST MEMORY this reminds me of?	What other SELF TALK attends this?

What EMOTION & BODY SENSATIONS do I feel/notice?

Where is this felt?

Size? Shape? Edges?

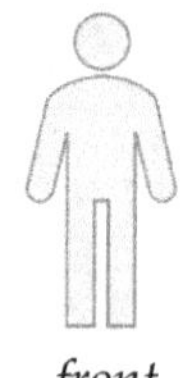 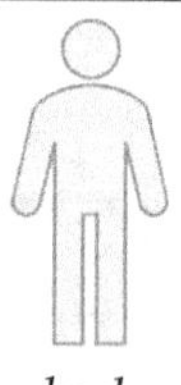

front   *back*

Intensity of Emotion BEFORE tapping:

1 2 3 4 5 6 7 8 9 10   Low – Medium – High

SET UP STATEMENT: 3x's at side of hand

"Even though

,*I deeply and completely accept myself"

Self-Acceptance Phrase

REMINDER PHRASE: at all other points

"This   in my

CHECK INTENSITY OF EMOTION: check after each round

Set Up for Additional Tapping as needed

"Even though ***I have some remaining*** _________, I deeply and completely accept myself."

"This ***remaining*** _______.

NOTES: ____

____

____

____

____

____

____

____

____

Date____________

<table><tr><td>

THE PROBLEM's "MOVIE TITLE"

</td></tr></table>

<table><tr><td>

THE NEGATIVE BELIEF/SELF-TALK:

</td></tr><tr><td>

Rate it: 1-100 (1= least intense, 100 = most intense)

</td></tr></table>

CONSIDER THE DETAILS (past/present/future):

WHAT event/condition happened?	WHEN did it start?
WHO was/will be involved?	WHAT was/is going on?
WHERE did/will it happen?	WHY did/will it happen?
WHEN did/will it happen?	HOW did/will it happen?

What does this REMIND me of?	What OTHER ISSUES came up?
What is the EARLIEST MEMORY this reminds me of?	What other SELF TALK attends this?

What EMOTION & BODY SENSATIONS do I feel/notice?

Where is this felt?

Size? Shape? Edges?

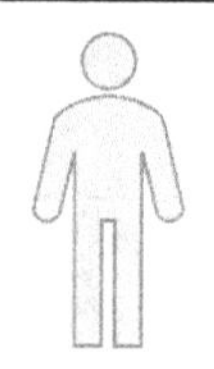 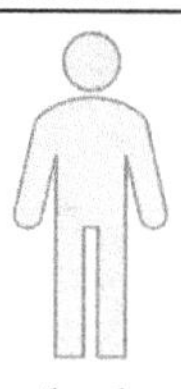

front   *back*

Intensity of Emotion BEFORE tapping:

1 2 3 4 5 6 7 8 9 10   Low – Medium – High

SET UP STATEMENT: 3x's at side of hand

> "Even though
>
>
>
>
>
> ,*I deeply and completely accept myself"

Self-Acceptance Phrase

REMINDER PHRASE: at all other points

> "This   in my

CHECK INTENSITY OF EMOTION: check after each round

Set Up for Additional Tapping as needed

"Even though *I have some remaining* _________, I deeply and completely accept myself."

"This *remaining* _______.

NOTES:
____

____

____

____

____

____

____

____

____

Date___________

THE PROBLEM's "MOVIE TITLE"

THE NEGATIVE BELIEF/SELF-TALK:

Rate it: 1-100 (1= least intense, 100 = most intense)

CONSIDER THE DETAILS (past/present/future):

WHAT event/condition happened?	WHEN did it start?
WHO was/will be involved?	WHAT was/is going on?
WHERE did/will it happen?	WHY did/will it happen?
WHEN did/will it happen?	HOW did/will it happen?

What does this REMIND me of?	What OTHER ISSUES came up?
What is the EARLIEST MEMORY this reminds me of?	What other SELF TALK attends this?

What EMOTION & BODY SENSATIONS do I feel/notice?

Where is this felt?

Size? Shape? Edges?

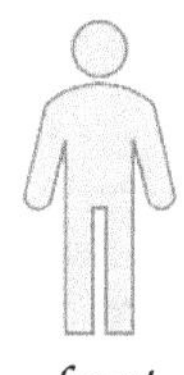 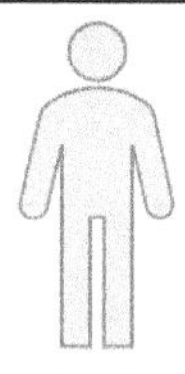

front   *back*

Intensity of Emotion BEFORE tapping:

1 2 3 4 5 6 7 8 9 10   Low – Medium – High

SET UP STATEMENT: 3x's at side of hand

"Even though

,*I deeply and completely accept myself"

Self-Acceptance Phrase

REMINDER PHRASE: at all other points

"This   in my

CHECK INTENSITY OF EMOTION: check after each round

Set Up for Additional Tapping as needed

"Even though ***I have some remaining*** ________, I deeply and completely accept myself."

"This ***remaining*** ______.

NOTES: ____

____

____

____

____

____

____

____

____

Date____________

THE PROBLEM's "MOVIE TITLE"

THE NEGATIVE BELIEF/SELF-TALK:

Rate it: 1-100 (1= least intense, 100 = most intense)

CONSIDER THE DETAILS (past/present/future):

WHAT event/condition happened?	WHEN did it start?
WHO was/will be involved?	WHAT was/is going on?
WHERE did/will it happen?	WHY did/will it happen?
WHEN did/will it happen?	HOW did/will it happen?

What does this REMIND me of?	What OTHER ISSUES came up?
What is the EARLIEST MEMORY this reminds me of?	What other SELF TALK attends this?

What EMOTION & BODY SENSATIONS do I feel/notice?

Where is this felt?

Size? Shape? Edges?

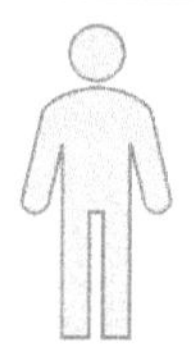

front

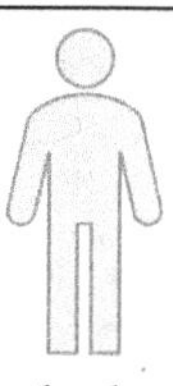

back

Intensity of Emotion BEFORE tapping:

1 2 3 4 5 6 7 8 9 10   Low – Medium – High

SET UP STATEMENT: 3x's at side of hand

> "Even though
>
>
>
>
>
>
> ,*I deeply and completely accept myself"

Self-Acceptance Phrase

REMINDER PHRASE: at all other points

> "This   in my

CHECK INTENSITY OF EMOTION: check after each round

Set Up for Additional Tapping as needed

"Even though *I have some remaining* __________, I deeply and completely accept myself."

"This *remaining* _______.

NOTES: ____

____

____

____

____

____

____

____

Date___________

THE PROBLEM's "MOVIE TITLE"

THE NEGATIVE BELIEF/SELF-TALK:

Rate it: 1-100 (1= least intense, 100 = most intense)

CONSIDER THE DETAILS (past/present/future):

WHAT event/condition happened?	WHEN did it start?
WHO was/will be involved?	WHAT was/is going on?
WHERE did/will it happen?	WHY did/will it happen?
WHEN did/will it happen?	HOW did/will it happen?

What does this REMIND me of?	What OTHER ISSUES came up?
What is the EARLIEST MEMORY this reminds me of?	What other SELF TALK attends this?

What EMOTION & BODY SENSATIONS do I feel/notice?

Where is this felt?

Size? Shape? Edges?

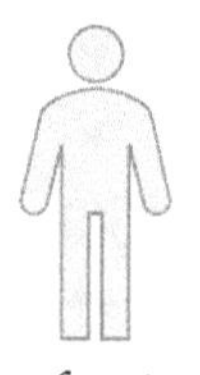 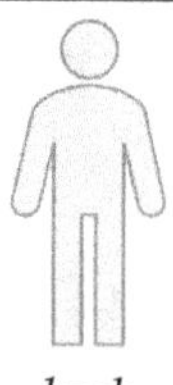

front   *back*

Intensity of Emotion BEFORE tapping:

1 2 3 4 5 6 7 8 9 10   Low – Medium – High

SET UP STATEMENT: 3x's at side of hand

"Even though

,*I deeply and completely accept myself"

*Self-Acceptance Phrase

REMINDER PHRASE: at all other points

"This   in my

CHECK INTENSITY OF EMOTION: check after each round

Set Up for Additional Tapping as needed

"Even though *I have some remaining* _________, I deeply and completely accept myself."

"This *remaining* _______.

NOTES: ____

____

____

____

____

____

____

____

____

Date___________

THE PROBLEM's "MOVIE TITLE"

THE NEGATIVE BELIEF/SELF-TALK:

Rate it: 1-100 (1= least intense, 100 = most intense)

CONSIDER THE DETAILS (past/present/future):

WHAT event/condition happened?	WHEN did it start?
WHO was/will be involved?	WHAT was/is going on?
WHERE did/will it happen?	WHY did/will it happen?
WHEN did/will it happen?	HOW did/will it happen?

What does this REMIND me of?	What OTHER ISSUES came up?
What is the EARLIEST MEMORY this reminds me of?	What other SELF TALK attends this?

What EMOTION & BODY SENSATIONS do I feel/notice?

Where is this felt?

Size? Shape? Edges?

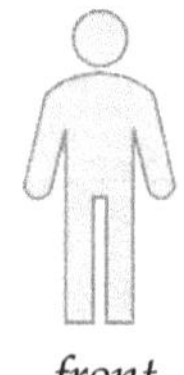 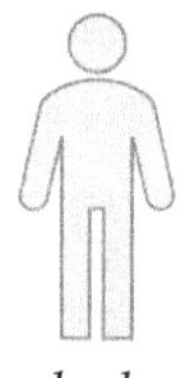

front *back*

Intensity of Emotion BEFORE tapping:

1 2 3 4 5 6 7 8 9 10   Low – Medium – High

SET UP STATEMENT: 3x's at side of hand

"Even though

,*I deeply and completely accept myself"

Self-Acceptance Phrase

REMINDER PHRASE: at all other points

"This   in my

CHECK INTENSITY OF EMOTION: check after each round

Set Up for Additional Tapping as needed

"Even though *I have some remaining* __________, I deeply and completely accept myself."

"This *remaining* _______.

NOTES: ____

____

____

____

____

____

____

____

____

Date_____________

THE PROBLEM's "MOVIE TITLE"

THE NEGATIVE BELIEF/SELF-TALK:

Rate it: 1-100 (1= least intense, 100 = most intense)

CONSIDER THE DETAILS (past/present/future):

WHAT event/condition happened?	WHEN did it start?
WHO was/will be involved?	WHAT was/is going on?
WHERE did/will it happen?	WHY did/will it happen?
WHEN did/will it happen?	HOW did/will it happen?

What does this REMIND me of?	What OTHER ISSUES came up?
What is the EARLIEST MEMORY this reminds me of?	What other SELF TALK attends this?

What EMOTION & BODY SENSATIONS do I feel/notice?

Where is this felt?

Size? Shape? Edges?

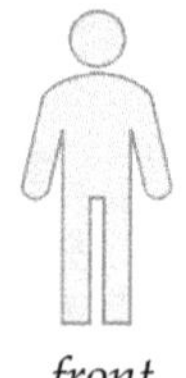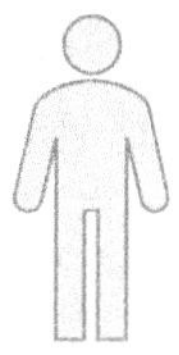

front   *back*

Intensity of Emotion BEFORE tapping:

1 2 3 4 5 6 7 8 9 10   Low – Medium – High

SET UP STATEMENT: 3x's at side of hand

"Even though

,*I deeply and completely accept myself"

Self-Acceptance Phrase

REMINDER PHRASE: at all other points

"This   in my

CHECK INTENSITY OF EMOTION: check after each round

Set Up for Additional Tapping as needed

"Even though *I have some remaining* _________, I deeply and completely accept myself."

"This *remaining* _______.

NOTES: ____

____

____

____

____

____

____

____

Date___________

<table>
<tr><td>

THE PROBLEM's "MOVIE TITLE"

</td></tr>
</table>

<table>
<tr><td>

THE NEGATIVE BELIEF/SELF-TALK:

Rate it: 1-100 (1= least intense, 100 = most intense)

</td></tr>
</table>

<table>
<tr><td colspan="2">

CONSIDER THE DETAILS (past/present/future):

</td></tr>
<tr><td>

WHAT event/condition happened?

WHO was/will be involved?

WHERE did/will it happen?

WHEN did/will it happen?

</td><td>

WHEN did it start?

WHAT was/is going on?

WHY did/will it happen?

HOW did/will it happen?

</td></tr>
<tr><td>

What does this REMIND me of?

What is the EARLIEST MEMORY this reminds me of?

</td><td>

What OTHER ISSUES came up?

What other SELF TALK attends this?

</td></tr>
</table>

<table>
<tr><td colspan="2">

What EMOTION & BODY SENSATIONS do I feel/notice?

</td></tr>
<tr><td>

Where is this felt?

Size? Shape? Edges?

</td><td>

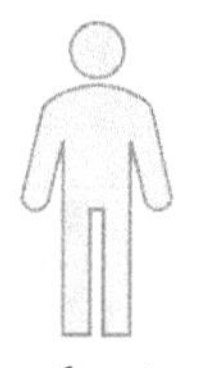 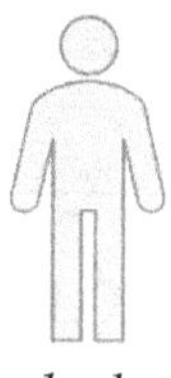

front　*back*

</td></tr>
<tr><td colspan="2">

Intensity of Emotion BEFORE tapping:

1 2 3 4 5 6 7 8 9 10   Low – Medium – High

</td></tr>
</table>

SET UP STATEMENT: 3x's at side of hand

"Even though

,*I deeply and completely accept myself"

Self-Acceptance Phrase

REMINDER PHRASE: at all other points

"This   in my

CHECK INTENSITY OF EMOTION: check after each round

Set Up for Additional Tapping as needed

"Even though *I have some remaining* _________, I deeply and completely accept myself."

"This *remaining* _______.

NOTES: ____

____

____

____

____

____

____

____

____

Date___________

<table>
<tr><td>THE PROBLEM's "MOVIE TITLE"</td></tr>
</table>

<table>
<tr><td>THE NEGATIVE BELIEF/SELF-TALK:</td></tr>
<tr><td>Rate it: 1-100 (1= least intense, 100 = most intense)</td></tr>
</table>

CONSIDER THE DETAILS (past/present/future):

WHAT event/condition happened?	WHEN did it start?
WHO was/will be involved?	WHAT was/is going on?
WHERE did/will it happen?	WHY did/will it happen?
WHEN did/will it happen?	HOW did/will it happen?

What does this REMIND me of?	What OTHER ISSUES came up?
What is the EARLIEST MEMORY this reminds me of?	What other SELF TALK attends this?

What EMOTION & BODY SENSATIONS do I feel/notice?

Where is this felt?

Size? Shape? Edges?

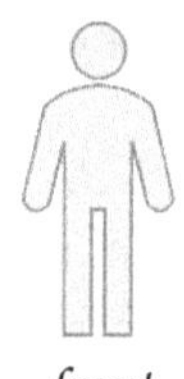

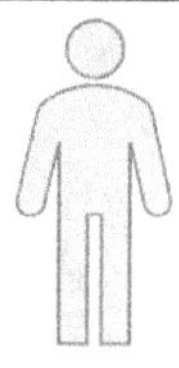

Intensity of Emotion BEFORE tapping:

1 2 3 4 5 6 7 8 9 10   Low – Medium – High

SET UP STATEMENT: 3x's at side of hand

"Even though

,*I deeply and completely accept myself"

*Self-Acceptance Phrase

REMINDER PHRASE: at all other points

"This   in my

CHECK INTENSITY OF EMOTION: check after each round

Set Up for Additional Tapping as needed

"Even though *I have some remaining* ________, I deeply and completely accept myself."

"This *remaining* ______.

NOTES: ____

____

____

____

____

____

____

____

____

Date____________

THE PROBLEM's "MOVIE TITLE"

THE NEGATIVE BELIEF/SELF-TALK:
Rate it: 1-100 (1= least intense, 100 = most intense)

CONSIDER THE DETAILS (past/present/future):

WHAT event/condition happened?	WHEN did it start?
WHO was/will be involved?	WHAT was/is going on?
WHERE did/will it happen?	WHY did/will it happen?
WHEN did/will it happen?	HOW did/will it happen?

What does this REMIND me of?	What OTHER ISSUES came up?
What is the EARLIEST MEMORY this reminds me of?	What other SELF TALK attends this?

What EMOTION & BODY SENSATIONS do I feel/notice?

Where is this felt?

Size? Shape? Edges?

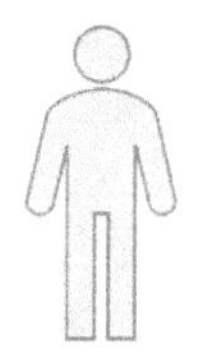
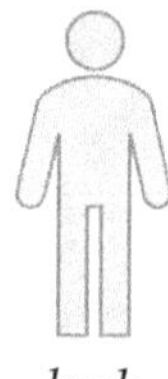

front   *back*

Intensity of Emotion BEFORE tapping:

1 2 3 4 5 6 7 8 9 10   Low – Medium – High

SET UP STATEMENT: 3x's at side of hand

"Even though

,*I deeply and completely accept myself"

**Self-Acceptance Phrase*

REMINDER PHRASE: at all other points

"This   in my

CHECK INTENSITY OF EMOTION: check after each round

Set Up for Additional Tapping as needed

"Even though *I have some remaining* __________, I deeply and completely accept myself."

"This *remaining* _______.

NOTES: ____

____

____

____

____

____

____

____

____

Date___________

THE PROBLEM's "MOVIE TITLE"

THE NEGATIVE BELIEF/SELF-TALK:

Rate it: 1-100 (1= least intense, 100 = most intense)

CONSIDER THE DETAILS (past/present/future):

WHAT event/condition happened?   WHEN did it start?

WHO was/will be involved?   WHAT was/is going on?

WHERE did/will it happen?   WHY did/will it happen?

WHEN did/will it happen?   HOW did/will it happen?

What does this REMIND me of?   What OTHER ISSUES came up?

What is the EARLIEST MEMORY   What other SELF TALK attends
this reminds me of?   this?

What EMOTION & BODY SENSATIONS do I feel/notice?

Where is this felt?

Size? Shape? Edges?

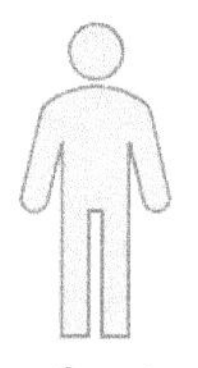 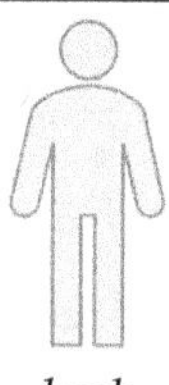

front   *back*

Intensity of Emotion BEFORE tapping:

1 2 3 4 5 6 7 8 9 10   Low – Medium – High

SET UP STATEMENT: 3x's at side of hand

"Even though

,*I deeply and completely accept myself"

Self-Acceptance Phrase

REMINDER PHRASE: at all other points

"This   in my

CHECK INTENSITY OF EMOTION: check after each round

Set Up for Additional Tapping as needed

"Even though *I have some remaining* _________, I deeply and completely accept myself."

"This *remaining* _______.

NOTES: _______________________________________

____

____

____

____

____

____

____

____

Date____________

<table>
<tr><td>

THE PROBLEM's "MOVIE TITLE"

</td></tr>
</table>

<table>
<tr><td>

THE NEGATIVE BELIEF/SELF-TALK:

Rate it: 1-100 (1= least intense, 100 = most intense)

</td></tr>
</table>

<table>
<tr><td colspan="2">

CONSIDER THE DETAILS (past/present/future):

</td></tr>
<tr><td>

WHAT event/condition happened?

WHO was/will be involved?

WHERE did/will it happen?

WHEN did/will it happen?

</td><td>

WHEN did it start?

WHAT was/is going on?

WHY did/will it happen?

HOW did/will it happen?

</td></tr>
<tr><td>

What does this REMIND me of?

What is the EARLIEST MEMORY this reminds me of?

</td><td>

What OTHER ISSUES came up?

What other SELF TALK attends this?

</td></tr>
</table>

<table>
<tr><td colspan="2">

What EMOTION & BODY SENSATIONS do I feel/notice?

</td></tr>
<tr><td>

Where is this felt?

Size? Shape? Edges?

</td><td>

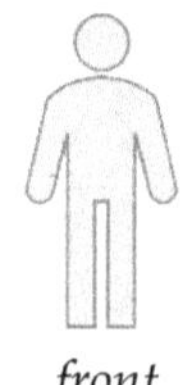 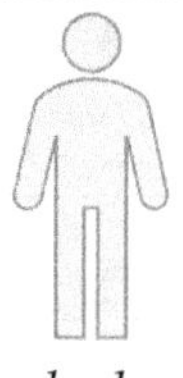

front   *back*

</td></tr>
<tr><td colspan="2">

Intensity of Emotion BEFORE tapping:

1 2 3 4 5 6 7 8 9 10   Low – Medium – High

</td></tr>
</table>

SET UP STATEMENT: 3x's at side of hand

"Even though

,*I deeply and completely accept myself"

*Self-Acceptance Phrase

REMINDER PHRASE: at all other points

"This   in my

CHECK INTENSITY OF EMOTION: check after each round

Set Up for Additional Tapping as needed

"Even though *I have some remaining* _________, I deeply and completely accept myself."

"This *remaining* _______.

NOTES: _______________________________________

____

____

____

____

____

____

____

____

Date_____________

THE PROBLEM's "MOVIE TITLE"

THE NEGATIVE BELIEF/SELF-TALK:

Rate it: 1-100 (1= least intense, 100 = most intense)

CONSIDER THE DETAILS (past/present/future):

WHAT event/condition happened?	WHEN did it start?
WHO was/will be involved?	WHAT was/is going on?
WHERE did/will it happen?	WHY did/will it happen?
WHEN did/will it happen?	HOW did/will it happen?

What does this REMIND me of?	What OTHER ISSUES came up?
What is the EARLIEST MEMORY this reminds me of?	What other SELF TALK attends this?

What EMOTION & BODY SENSATIONS do I feel/notice?

Where is this felt?

Size? Shape? Edges?

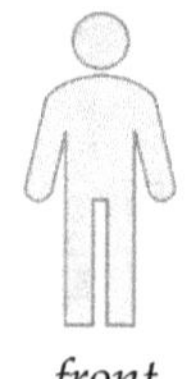 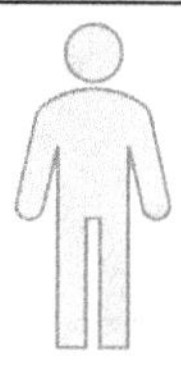

front   *back*

Intensity of Emotion BEFORE tapping:

1 2 3 4 5 6 7 8 9 10   Low – Medium – High

SET UP STATEMENT: 3x's at side of hand

> "Even though
>
>
>
>
> ,*I deeply and completely accept myself"

Self-Acceptance Phrase

REMINDER PHRASE: at all other points

> "This   in my

CHECK INTENSITY OF EMOTION: check after each round

Set Up for Additional Tapping as needed

"Even though *I have some remaining* __________, I deeply and completely accept myself."

"This *remaining* _______.

NOTES: ____

____

____

____

____

____

____

____

Date___________

<table>
<tr><td>

THE PROBLEM's "MOVIE TITLE"

</td></tr>
</table>

<table>
<tr><td>

THE NEGATIVE BELIEF/SELF-TALK:

Rate it: 1-100 (1= least intense, 100 = most intense)

</td></tr>
</table>

CONSIDER THE DETAILS (past/present/future):

WHAT event/condition happened?	WHEN did it start?
WHO was/will be involved?	WHAT was/is going on?
WHERE did/will it happen?	WHY did/will it happen?
WHEN did/will it happen?	HOW did/will it happen?

What does this REMIND me of?	What OTHER ISSUES came up?
What is the EARLIEST MEMORY this reminds me of?	What other SELF TALK attends this?

What EMOTION & BODY SENSATIONS do I feel/notice?

Where is this felt?

Size? Shape? Edges?

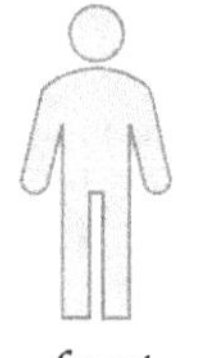 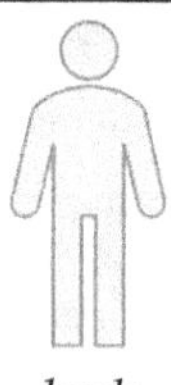

front   *back*

Intensity of Emotion BEFORE tapping:

1 2 3 4 5 6 7 8 9 10   Low – Medium – High

SET UP STATEMENT: 3x's at side of hand

"Even though

,*I deeply and completely accept myself"

Self-Acceptance Phrase

REMINDER PHRASE: at all other points

"This   in my

CHECK INTENSITY OF EMOTION: check after each round

Set Up for Additional Tapping as needed

"Even though ***I have some remaining*** _________, I deeply and completely accept myself."

"This ***remaining*** _______.

NOTES: ____

____

____

____

____

____

____

____

____

Date_____________

<table>
<tr><td>

THE PROBLEM's "MOVIE TITLE"

</td></tr>
</table>

<table>
<tr><td>

THE NEGATIVE BELIEF/SELF-TALK:

</td></tr>
<tr><td>

Rate it: 1-100 (1= least intense, 100 = most intense)

</td></tr>
</table>

<table>
<tr><td colspan="2">

CONSIDER THE DETAILS (past/present/future):

</td></tr>
<tr><td>

WHAT event/condition happened?

WHO was/will be involved?

WHERE did/will it happen?

WHEN did/will it happen?

</td><td>

WHEN did it start?

WHAT was/is going on?

WHY did/will it happen?

HOW did/will it happen?

</td></tr>
<tr><td>

What does this REMIND me of?

What is the EARLIEST MEMORY this reminds me of?

</td><td>

What OTHER ISSUES came up?

What other SELF TALK attends this?

</td></tr>
</table>

<table>
<tr><td colspan="2">

What EMOTION & BODY SENSATIONS do I feel/notice?

</td></tr>
<tr><td>

Where is this felt?

Size? Shape? Edges?

</td><td>

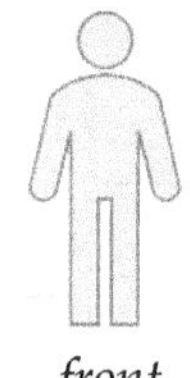 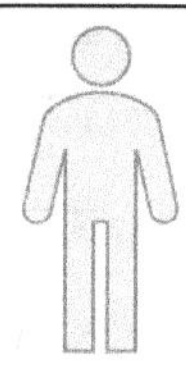

front   *back*

</td></tr>
<tr><td colspan="2">

Intensity of Emotion BEFORE tapping:

1 2 3 4 5 6 7 8 9 10   Low – Medium – High

</td></tr>
</table>

SET UP STATEMENT: 3x's at side of hand

"Even though

,*I deeply and completely accept myself"

*Self-Acceptance Phrase

REMINDER PHRASE: at all other points

"This   in my

CHECK INTENSITY OF EMOTION: check after each round

Set Up for Additional Tapping as needed

"Even though *I have some remaining* __________, I deeply and completely accept myself."

"This *remaining* _______.

NOTES:

____

____

____

____

____

____

____

____

Date___________

<table>
<tr><td>

THE PROBLEM's "MOVIE TITLE"

</td></tr>
</table>

<table>
<tr><td>

THE NEGATIVE BELIEF/SELF-TALK:

</td></tr>
<tr><td>

Rate it: 1-100 (1= least intense, 100 = most intense)

</td></tr>
</table>

<table>
<tr><td colspan="2">

CONSIDER THE DETAILS (past/present/future):

</td></tr>
<tr><td>

WHAT event/condition happened?

WHO was/will be involved?

WHERE did/will it happen?

WHEN did/will it happen?

</td><td>

WHEN did it start?

WHAT was/is going on?

WHY did/will it happen?

HOW did/will it happen?

</td></tr>
<tr><td>

What does this REMIND me of?

What is the EARLIEST MEMORY this reminds me of?

</td><td>

What OTHER ISSUES came up?

What other SELF TALK attends this?

</td></tr>
</table>

<table>
<tr><td colspan="2">

What EMOTION & BODY SENSATIONS do I feel/notice?

</td></tr>
<tr><td>

Where is this felt?

Size? Shape? Edges?

</td><td>

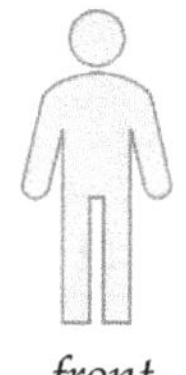 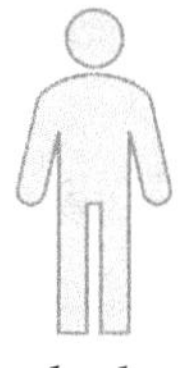

front   *back*

</td></tr>
<tr><td colspan="2">

Intensity of Emotion BEFORE tapping:

1 2 3 4 5 6 7 8 9 10   Low – Medium – High

</td></tr>
</table>

SET UP STATEMENT: 3x's at side of hand

"Even though

,*I deeply and completely accept myself"

*Self-Acceptance Phrase

REMINDER PHRASE: at all other points

"This   in my

CHECK INTENSITY OF EMOTION: check after each round

Set Up for Additional Tapping as needed

"Even though ***I have some remaining*** _________, I deeply and completely accept myself."

"This ***remaining*** _______.

NOTES: ____

____

____

____

____

____

____

____

____

Date___________

THE PROBLEM's "MOVIE TITLE"

THE NEGATIVE BELIEF/SELF-TALK:

Rate it: 1-100 (1= least intense, 100 = most intense)

CONSIDER THE DETAILS (past/present/future):

WHAT event/condition happened?	WHEN did it start?
WHO was/will be involved?	WHAT was/is going on?
WHERE did/will it happen?	WHY did/will it happen?
WHEN did/will it happen?	HOW did/will it happen?

What does this REMIND me of?	What OTHER ISSUES came up?
What is the EARLIEST MEMORY this reminds me of?	What other SELF TALK attends this?

What EMOTION & BODY SENSATIONS do I feel/notice?

Where is this felt?

Size? Shape? Edges?

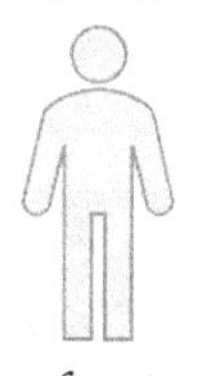 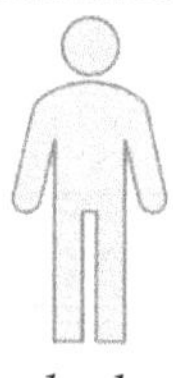

front   *back*

Intensity of Emotion BEFORE tapping:

1 2 3 4 5 6 7 8 9 10   Low – Medium – High

SET UP STATEMENT: 3x's at side of hand

"Even though

,*I deeply and completely accept myself"

**Self-Acceptance Phrase*

REMINDER PHRASE: at all other points

"This   in my

CHECK INTENSITY OF EMOTION: check after each round

Set Up for Additional Tapping as needed

"Even though *I have some remaining* _________, I deeply and completely accept myself."

"This *remaining* _______.

NOTES: ____

____

____

____

____

____

____

____

____

Date___________

THE PROBLEM's "MOVIE TITLE"

THE NEGATIVE BELIEF/SELF-TALK:

Rate it: 1-100 (1= least intense, 100 = most intense)

CONSIDER THE DETAILS (past/present/future):

WHAT event/condition happened?	WHEN did it start?
WHO was/will be involved?	WHAT was/is going on?
WHERE did/will it happen?	WHY did/will it happen?
WHEN did/will it happen?	HOW did/will it happen?

What does this REMIND me of?	What OTHER ISSUES came up?
What is the EARLIEST MEMORY this reminds me of?	What other SELF TALK attends this?

What EMOTION & BODY SENSATIONS do I feel/notice?

Where is this felt?
Size? Shape? Edges?

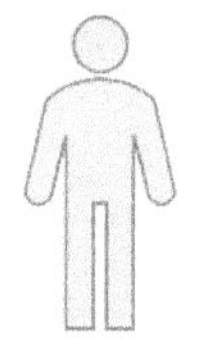 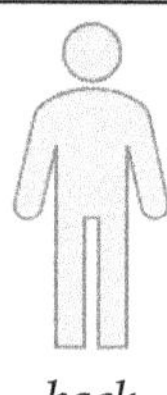

Intensity of Emotion BEFORE tapping:

1 2 3 4 5 6 7 8 9 10   Low – Medium – High

SET UP STATEMENT: 3x's at side of hand

"Even though

,*I deeply and completely accept myself"

*Self-Acceptance Phrase

REMINDER PHRASE: at all other points

"This   in my

CHECK INTENSITY OF EMOTION: check after each round

Set Up for Additional Tapping as needed

"Even though *I have some remaining* ________, I deeply and completely accept myself."

"This *remaining* ______.

NOTES:

Date___________

THE PROBLEM's "MOVIE TITLE"

THE NEGATIVE BELIEF/SELF-TALK:

Rate it: 1-100 (1= least intense, 100 = most intense)

CONSIDER THE DETAILS (past/present/future):

WHAT event/condition happened?	WHEN did it start?
WHO was/will be involved?	WHAT was/is going on?
WHERE did/will it happen?	WHY did/will it happen?
WHEN did/will it happen?	HOW did/will it happen?

What does this REMIND me of?	What OTHER ISSUES came up?
What is the EARLIEST MEMORY this reminds me of?	What other SELF TALK attends this?

What EMOTION & BODY SENSATIONS do I feel/notice?

Where is this felt?

Size? Shape? Edges?

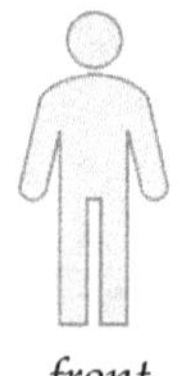 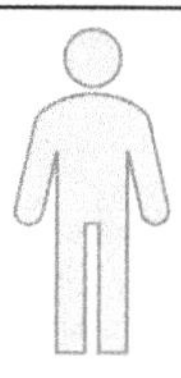

front   *back*

Intensity of Emotion BEFORE tapping:

1 2 3 4 5 6 7 8 9 10   Low – Medium – High

SET UP STATEMENT: 3x's at side of hand

"Even though

,*I deeply and completely accept myself"

Self-Acceptance Phrase

REMINDER PHRASE: at all other points

"This   in my

CHECK INTENSITY OF EMOTION: check after each round

Set Up for Additional Tapping as needed

"Even though *I have some remaining* __________, I deeply and completely accept myself."

"This *remaining* _______.

NOTES: ____

____

____

____

____

____

____

____

____

____

Date___________

<table>
<tr><td>

THE PROBLEM's "MOVIE TITLE"

</td></tr>
</table>

<table>
<tr><td>

THE NEGATIVE BELIEF/SELF-TALK:

Rate it: 1-100 (1= least intense, 100 = most intense)

</td></tr>
</table>

<table>
<tr><td colspan="2">

CONSIDER THE DETAILS (past/present/future):

</td></tr>
<tr><td>

WHAT event/condition happened?

WHO was/will be involved?

WHERE did/will it happen?

WHEN did/will it happen?

</td><td>

WHEN did it start?

WHAT was/is going on?

WHY did/will it happen?

HOW did/will it happen?

</td></tr>
<tr><td>

What does this REMIND me of?

What is the EARLIEST MEMORY this reminds me of?

</td><td>

What OTHER ISSUES came up?

What other SELF TALK attends this?

</td></tr>
</table>

<table>
<tr><td colspan="2">

What EMOTION & BODY SENSATIONS do I feel/notice?

</td></tr>
<tr><td>

Where is this felt?

Size? Shape? Edges?

</td><td>

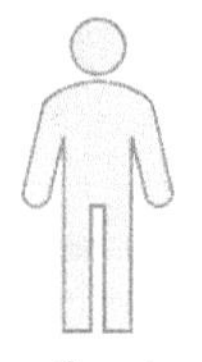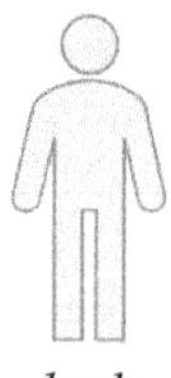

front   *back*

</td></tr>
<tr><td colspan="2">

Intensity of Emotion BEFORE tapping:

1 2 3 4 5 6 7 8 9 10   Low – Medium – High

</td></tr>
</table>

SET UP STATEMENT: 3x's at side of hand

"Even though

,*I deeply and completely accept myself"

Self-Acceptance Phrase

REMINDER PHRASE: at all other points

"This   in my

CHECK INTENSITY OF EMOTION: check after each round

Set Up for Additional Tapping as needed

"Even though *I have some remaining* _________, I deeply and completely accept myself."

"This *remaining* _______.

NOTES: _______________________________________

____

____

____

____

____

____

____

____

Date___________

THE PROBLEM's "MOVIE TITLE"

THE NEGATIVE BELIEF/SELF-TALK:
Rate it: 1-100 (1= least intense, 100 = most intense)

CONSIDER THE DETAILS (past/present/future):

WHAT event/condition happened?	WHEN did it start?
WHO was/will be involved?	WHAT was/is going on?
WHERE did/will it happen?	WHY did/will it happen?
WHEN did/will it happen?	HOW did/will it happen?

What does this REMIND me of?	What OTHER ISSUES came up?
What is the EARLIEST MEMORY this reminds me of?	What other SELF TALK attends this?

What EMOTION & BODY SENSATIONS do I feel/notice?

Where is this felt?

Size? Shape? Edges?

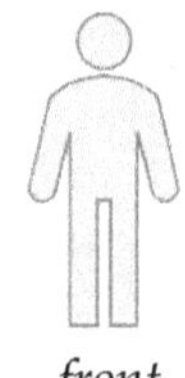
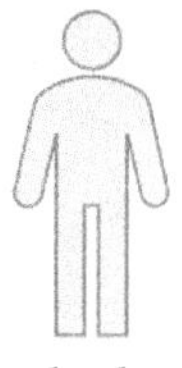

front   *back*

Intensity of Emotion BEFORE tapping:

1 2 3 4 5 6 7 8 9 10   Low – Medium – High

SET UP STATEMENT: 3x's at side of hand

> "Even though
>
>
>
>
> ,*I deeply and completely accept myself"

Self-Acceptance Phrase

REMINDER PHRASE: at all other points

"This   in my

CHECK INTENSITY OF EMOTION: check after each round

Set Up for Additional Tapping as needed

"Even though *I have some remaining* _________, I deeply and completely accept myself."

"This *remaining* _______.

NOTES: ____

____

____

____

____

____

____

____

____

Date___________

<table>
<tr><td>

THE PROBLEM's "MOVIE TITLE"

</td></tr>
</table>

<table>
<tr><td>

THE NEGATIVE BELIEF/SELF-TALK:

</td></tr>
<tr><td>

Rate it: 1-100 (1= least intense, 100 = most intense)

</td></tr>
</table>

CONSIDER THE DETAILS (past/present/future):

WHAT event/condition happened?	WHEN did it start?
WHO was/will be involved?	WHAT was/is going on?
WHERE did/will it happen?	WHY did/will it happen?
WHEN did/will it happen?	HOW did/will it happen?

What does this REMIND me of?	What OTHER ISSUES came up?
What is the EARLIEST MEMORY this reminds me of?	What other SELF TALK attends this?

What EMOTION & BODY SENSATIONS do I feel/notice?

Where is this felt?

Size? Shape? Edges?

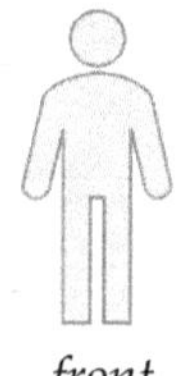
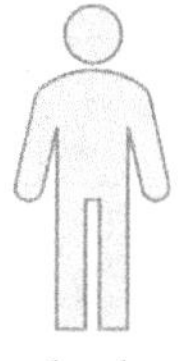

front   *back*

Intensity of Emotion BEFORE tapping:

1 2 3 4 5 6 7 8 9 10   Low – Medium – High

SET UP STATEMENT: 3x's at side of hand

"Even though

,*I deeply and completely accept myself"

Self-Acceptance Phrase

REMINDER PHRASE: at all other points

"This   in my

CHECK INTENSITY OF EMOTION: check after each round

Set Up for Additional Tapping as needed

"Even though **I have some remaining** __________, I deeply and completely accept myself."

"This **remaining** _______.

NOTES: ____

____

____

____

____

____

____

____

____

Date___________

THE PROBLEM's "MOVIE TITLE"

THE NEGATIVE BELIEF/SELF-TALK:

Rate it: 1-100 (1= least intense, 100 = most intense)

CONSIDER THE DETAILS (past/present/future):

WHAT event/condition happened?	WHEN did it start?
WHO was/will be involved?	WHAT was/is going on?
WHERE did/will it happen?	WHY did/will it happen?
WHEN did/will it happen?	HOW did/will it happen?

What does this REMIND me of?	What OTHER ISSUES came up?
What is the EARLIEST MEMORY this reminds me of?	What other SELF TALK attends this?

What EMOTION & BODY SENSATIONS do I feel/notice?

Where is this felt?

Size? Shape? Edges?

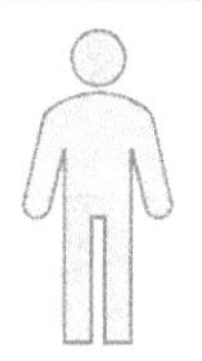 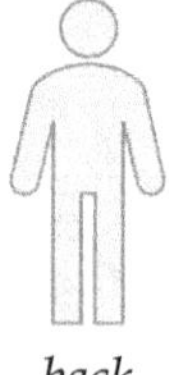

front   *back*

Intensity of Emotion BEFORE tapping:

1 2 3 4 5 6 7 8 9 10   Low – Medium – High

SET UP STATEMENT: 3x's at side of hand

"Even though

,*I deeply and completely accept myself"

*Self-Acceptance Phrase

REMINDER PHRASE: at all other points

"This   in my

CHECK INTENSITY OF EMOTION: check after each round

Set Up for Additional Tapping as needed

"Even though *I have some remaining* _________, I deeply and completely accept myself."

"This *remaining* _______.

NOTES: ____

____

____

____

____

____

____

____

Date____________

<table>
<tr><td>

THE PROBLEM's "MOVIE TITLE"

</td></tr>
</table>

<table>
<tr><td>

THE NEGATIVE BELIEF/SELF-TALK:

</td></tr>
<tr><td>

Rate it: 1-100 (1= least intense, 100 = most intense)

</td></tr>
</table>

CONSIDER THE DETAILS (past/present/future):

WHAT event/condition happened?	WHEN did it start?
WHO was/will be involved?	WHAT was/is going on?
WHERE did/will it happen?	WHY did/will it happen?
WHEN did/will it happen?	HOW did/will it happen?

What does this REMIND me of?	What OTHER ISSUES came up?
What is the EARLIEST MEMORY this reminds me of?	What other SELF TALK attends this?

What EMOTION & BODY SENSATIONS do I feel/notice?

Where is this felt?

Size? Shape? Edges?

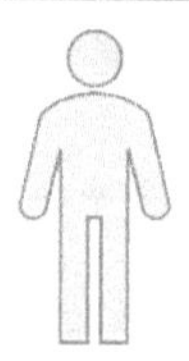 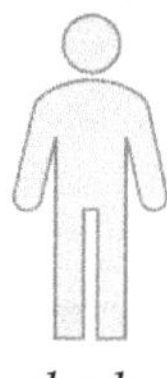

front   *back*

Intensity of Emotion BEFORE tapping:

1 2 3 4 5 6 7 8 9 10   Low – Medium – High

SET UP STATEMENT: 3x's at side of hand

> "Even though
>
>
>
>
>
> ,*I deeply and completely accept myself"

Self-Acceptance Phrase

REMINDER PHRASE: at all other points

> "This   in my

CHECK INTENSITY OF EMOTION: check after each round

Set Up for Additional Tapping as needed

"Even though *I have some remaining* _________, I deeply and completely accept myself."

"This *remaining* _______.

NOTES: _______________________________________

____

____

____

____

____

____

____

____

Date___________

<table>
<tr><td>THE PROBLEM's "MOVIE TITLE"</td></tr>
</table>

<table>
<tr><td>THE NEGATIVE BELIEF/SELF-TALK:</td></tr>
<tr><td>Rate it: 1-100 (1= least intense, 100 = most intense)</td></tr>
</table>

CONSIDER THE DETAILS (past/present/future):

WHAT event/condition happened?	WHEN did it start?
WHO was/will be involved?	WHAT was/is going on?
WHERE did/will it happen?	WHY did/will it happen?
WHEN did/will it happen?	HOW did/will it happen?

What does this REMIND me of?	What OTHER ISSUES came up?
What is the EARLIEST MEMORY this reminds me of?	What other SELF TALK attends this?

What EMOTION & BODY SENSATIONS do I feel/notice?

Where is this felt?

Size? Shape? Edges?

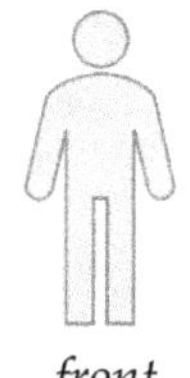
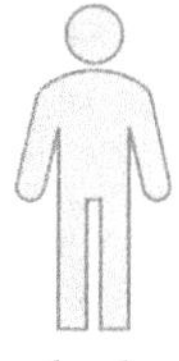

front   *back*

Intensity of Emotion BEFORE tapping:

1 2 3 4 5 6 7 8 9 10   Low – Medium – High

SET UP STATEMENT: 3x's at side of hand

"Even though

,*I deeply and completely accept myself"

Self-Acceptance Phrase

REMINDER PHRASE: at all other points

"This   in my

CHECK INTENSITY OF EMOTION: check after each round

Set Up for Additional Tapping as needed

"Even though *I have some remaining* _________, I deeply and completely accept myself."

"This *remaining* _______.

NOTES: _______________________________________

____

____

____

____

____

____

____

____

Date___________

<table>
<tr><td>

THE PROBLEM's "MOVIE TITLE"

</td></tr>
</table>

<table>
<tr><td>

THE NEGATIVE BELIEF/SELF-TALK:

</td></tr>
<tr><td>

Rate it: 1-100 (1= least intense, 100 = most intense)

</td></tr>
</table>

<table>
<tr><td colspan="2">

CONSIDER THE DETAILS (past/present/future):

</td></tr>
<tr><td>

WHAT event/condition happened?

WHO was/will be involved?

WHERE did/will it happen?

WHEN did/will it happen?

</td><td>

WHEN did it start?

WHAT was/is going on?

WHY did/will it happen?

HOW did/will it happen?

</td></tr>
<tr><td>

What does this REMIND me of?

What is the EARLIEST MEMORY this reminds me of?

</td><td>

What OTHER ISSUES came up?

What other SELF TALK attends this?

</td></tr>
</table>

<table>
<tr><td colspan="2">

What EMOTION & BODY SENSATIONS do I feel/notice?

</td></tr>
<tr><td>

Where is this felt?

Size? Shape? Edges?

</td><td>

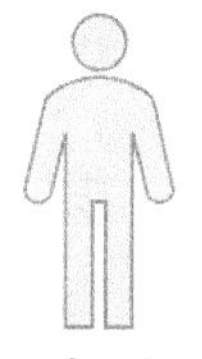 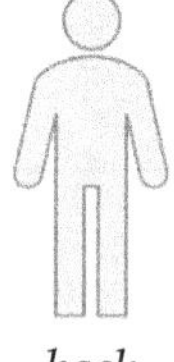

front   *back*

</td></tr>
<tr><td colspan="2">

Intensity of Emotion BEFORE tapping:

</td></tr>
<tr><td colspan="2">

1 2 3 4 5 6 7 8 9 10   Low – Medium – High

</td></tr>
</table>

SET UP STATEMENT: 3x's at side of hand

"Even though

,*I deeply and completely accept myself"

Self-Acceptance Phrase

REMINDER PHRASE: at all other points

"This   in my

CHECK INTENSITY OF EMOTION: check after each round

Set Up for Additional Tapping as needed

"Even though *I have some remaining* _________, I deeply and completely accept myself."

"This *remaining* _______.

NOTES: _______________________________________

____

____

____

____

____

____

____

____

____

Date___________

THE PROBLEM's "MOVIE TITLE"

THE NEGATIVE BELIEF/SELF-TALK:

Rate it: 1-100 (1= least intense, 100 = most intense)

CONSIDER THE DETAILS (past/present/future):

WHAT event/condition happened?	WHEN did it start?
WHO was/will be involved?	WHAT was/is going on?
WHERE did/will it happen?	WHY did/will it happen?
WHEN did/will it happen?	HOW did/will it happen?

What does this REMIND me of?	What OTHER ISSUES came up?
What is the EARLIEST MEMORY this reminds me of?	What other SELF TALK attends this?

What EMOTION & BODY SENSATIONS do I feel/notice?

Where is this felt?

Size? Shape? Edges?

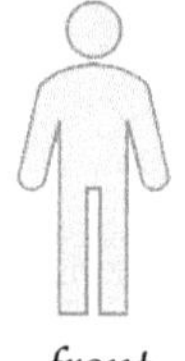 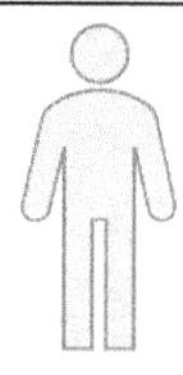

front   *back*

Intensity of Emotion BEFORE tapping:

1 2 3 4 5 6 7 8 9 10   Low – Medium – High

SET UP STATEMENT: 3x's at side of hand

> "Even though
>
>
>
>
>
> ,*I deeply and completely accept myself"

Self-Acceptance Phrase

REMINDER PHRASE: at all other points

> "This   in my

CHECK INTENSITY OF EMOTION: check after each round

Set Up for Additional Tapping as needed

"Even though *I have some remaining* _________, I deeply and completely accept myself."

"This *remaining* _______.

NOTES: ____

____

____

____

____

____

____

____

____

Date___________

THE PROBLEM's "MOVIE TITLE"

THE NEGATIVE BELIEF/SELF-TALK:

Rate it: 1-100 (1= least intense, 100 = most intense)

CONSIDER THE DETAILS (past/present/future):

WHAT event/condition happened?	WHEN did it start?
WHO was/will be involved?	WHAT was/is going on?
WHERE did/will it happen?	WHY did/will it happen?
WHEN did/will it happen?	HOW did/will it happen?

What does this REMIND me of?	What OTHER ISSUES came up?
What is the EARLIEST MEMORY this reminds me of?	What other SELF TALK attends this?

What EMOTION & BODY SENSATIONS do I feel/notice?

Where is this felt?

Size? Shape? Edges?

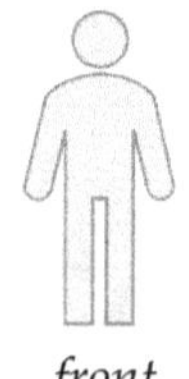 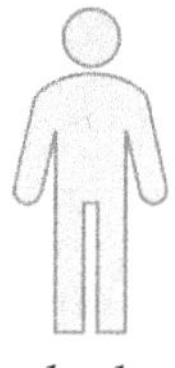

front　　*back*

Intensity of Emotion BEFORE tapping:

1 2 3 4 5 6 7 8 9 10   Low – Medium – High

SET UP STATEMENT: 3x's at side of hand

"Even though

,*I deeply and completely accept myself"

Self-Acceptance Phrase

REMINDER PHRASE: at all other points

"This   in my

CHECK INTENSITY OF EMOTION: check after each round

Set Up for Additional Tapping as needed

"Even though *I have some remaining* __________, I deeply and completely accept myself."

"This *remaining* _______.

NOTES: ____

____

____

____

____

____

____

____

____

Date___________

THE PROBLEM's "MOVIE TITLE"

THE NEGATIVE BELIEF/SELF-TALK:

Rate it: 1-100 (1= least intense, 100 = most intense)

CONSIDER THE DETAILS (past/present/future):

WHAT event/condition happened?	WHEN did it start?
WHO was/will be involved?	WHAT was/is going on?
WHERE did/will it happen?	WHY did/will it happen?
WHEN did/will it happen?	HOW did/will it happen?

What does this REMIND me of?	What OTHER ISSUES came up?
What is the EARLIEST MEMORY this reminds me of?	What other SELF TALK attends this?

What EMOTION & BODY SENSATIONS do I feel/notice?

Where is this felt?

Size? Shape? Edges?

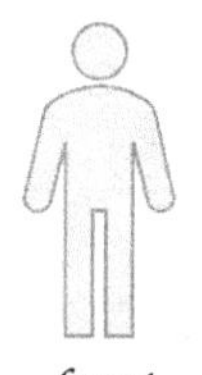 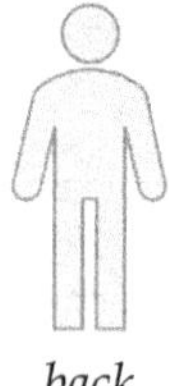

front   *back*

Intensity of Emotion BEFORE tapping:

1 2 3 4 5 6 7 8 9 10   Low – Medium – High

SET UP STATEMENT: 3x's at side of hand

"Even though

,*I deeply and completely accept myself"

Self-Acceptance Phrase

REMINDER PHRASE: at all other points

"This   in my

CHECK INTENSITY OF EMOTION: check after each round

Set Up for Additional Tapping as needed

"Even though *I have some remaining* _________, I deeply and completely accept myself."

"This *remaining* _______.

NOTES: ____

____

____

____

____

____

____

____

____

Date___________

<table>
<tr><td>THE PROBLEM's "MOVIE TITLE"</td></tr>
</table>

<table>
<tr><td>THE NEGATIVE BELIEF/SELF-TALK:</td></tr>
<tr><td>Rate it: 1-100 (1= least intense, 100 = most intense)</td></tr>
</table>

<table>
<tr><td colspan="2">CONSIDER THE DETAILS (past/present/future):</td></tr>
<tr><td>WHAT event/condition happened?</td><td>WHEN did it start?</td></tr>
<tr><td>WHO was/will be involved?</td><td>WHAT was/is going on?</td></tr>
<tr><td>WHERE did/will it happen?</td><td>WHY did/will it happen?</td></tr>
<tr><td>WHEN did/will it happen?</td><td>HOW did/will it happen?</td></tr>
<tr><td>What does this REMIND me of?
What is the EARLIEST MEMORY this reminds me of?</td><td>What OTHER ISSUES came up?
What other SELF TALK attends this?</td></tr>
</table>

<table>
<tr><td colspan="2">What EMOTION & BODY SENSATIONS do I feel/notice?</td></tr>
<tr><td>Where is this felt?
Size? Shape? Edges?</td><td>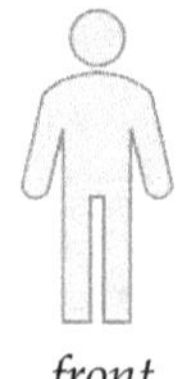 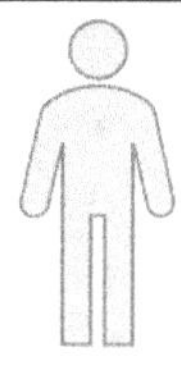
front   back</td></tr>
<tr><td colspan="2">Intensity of Emotion BEFORE tapping:</td></tr>
<tr><td>1 2 3 4 5 6 7 8 9 10</td><td>Low – Medium – High</td></tr>
</table>

SET UP STATEMENT: 3x's at side of hand

"Even though

,*I deeply and completely accept myself"

*Self-Acceptance Phrase

REMINDER PHRASE: at all other points

"This   in my

CHECK INTENSITY OF EMOTION: check after each round

Set Up for Additional Tapping as needed

"Even though *I have some remaining* _________, I deeply and completely accept myself."

"This *remaining* _______.

NOTES: ____

____

____

____

____

____

____

____

____

Date___________

THE PROBLEM's "MOVIE TITLE"

THE NEGATIVE BELIEF/SELF-TALK:

Rate it: 1-100 (1= least intense, 100 = most intense)

CONSIDER THE DETAILS (past/present/future):

WHAT event/condition happened?	WHEN did it start?
WHO was/will be involved?	WHAT was/is going on?
WHERE did/will it happen?	WHY did/will it happen?
WHEN did/will it happen?	HOW did/will it happen?

What does this REMIND me of?	What OTHER ISSUES came up?
What is the EARLIEST MEMORY this reminds me of?	What other SELF TALK attends this?

What EMOTION & BODY SENSATIONS do I feel/notice?

Where is this felt?

Size? Shape? Edges?

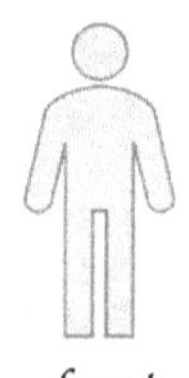

front

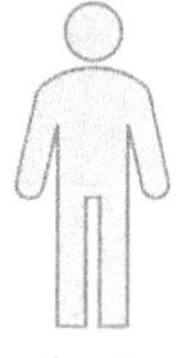

back

Intensity of Emotion BEFORE tapping:

1 2 3 4 5 6 7 8 9 10   Low – Medium – High

SET UP STATEMENT: 3x's at side of hand

"Even though

,*I deeply and completely accept myself"

Self-Acceptance Phrase

REMINDER PHRASE: at all other points

"This   in my

CHECK INTENSITY OF EMOTION: check after each round

Set Up for Additional Tapping as needed

"Even though **I have some remaining** _________, I deeply and completely accept myself."

"This **remaining** _______.

NOTES: _______________________________

____

____

____

____

____

____

____

____

Date___________

<table>
<tr><td>THE PROBLEM's "MOVIE TITLE"</td></tr>
</table>

<table>
<tr><td>THE NEGATIVE BELIEF/SELF-TALK:</td></tr>
<tr><td>Rate it: 1-100 (1= least intense, 100 = most intense)</td></tr>
</table>

CONSIDER THE DETAILS (past/present/future):

WHAT event/condition happened?	WHEN did it start?
WHO was/will be involved?	WHAT was/is going on?
WHERE did/will it happen?	WHY did/will it happen?
WHEN did/will it happen?	HOW did/will it happen?

What does this REMIND me of?	What OTHER ISSUES came up?
What is the EARLIEST MEMORY this reminds me of?	What other SELF TALK attends this?

What EMOTION & BODY SENSATIONS do I feel/notice?

Where is this felt?

Size? Shape? Edges?

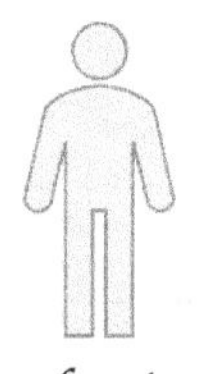 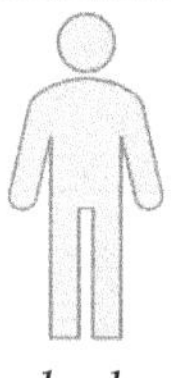

front   *back*

Intensity of Emotion BEFORE tapping:

1 2 3 4 5 6 7 8 9 10   Low – Medium – High

SET UP STATEMENT: 3x's at side of hand

"Even though

,*I deeply and completely accept myself"

*Self-Acceptance Phrase

REMINDER PHRASE: at all other points

"This   in my

CHECK INTENSITY OF EMOTION: check after each round

Set Up for Additional Tapping as needed

"Even though *I have some remaining* ________, I deeply and completely accept myself."

"This *remaining* ______.

NOTES: _____________________________________

____

____

____

____

____

____

____

Date___________

<table>
<tr><td>

THE PROBLEM's "MOVIE TITLE"

</td></tr>
</table>

<table>
<tr><td>

THE NEGATIVE BELIEF/SELF-TALK:

</td></tr>
<tr><td>

Rate it: 1-100 (1= least intense, 100 = most intense)

</td></tr>
</table>

<table>
<tr><td colspan="2">

CONSIDER THE DETAILS (past/present/future):

</td></tr>
<tr><td>

WHAT event/condition happened?

WHO was/will be involved?

WHERE did/will it happen?

WHEN did/will it happen?

</td><td>

WHEN did it start?

WHAT was/is going on?

WHY did/will it happen?

HOW did/will it happen?

</td></tr>
<tr><td>

What does this REMIND me of?

What is the EARLIEST MEMORY this reminds me of?

</td><td>

What OTHER ISSUES came up?

What other SELF TALK attends this?

</td></tr>
</table>

<table>
<tr><td colspan="2">

What EMOTION & BODY SENSATIONS do I feel/notice?

</td></tr>
<tr><td>

Where is this felt?

Size? Shape? Edges?

</td><td>

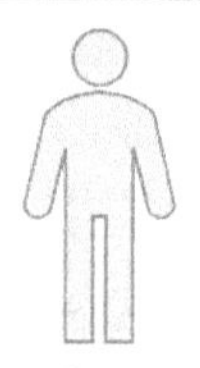 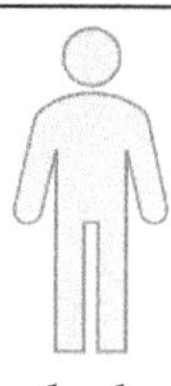

front   *back*

</td></tr>
</table>

<table>
<tr><td colspan="2">

Intensity of Emotion BEFORE tapping:

</td></tr>
<tr><td>

1 2 3 4 5 6 7 8 9 10

</td><td>

Low – Medium – High

</td></tr>
</table>

SET UP STATEMENT: 3x's at side of hand

"Even though

                              ,*I deeply and completely accept myself"

Self-Acceptance Phrase

REMINDER PHRASE: at all other points

"This   in my

CHECK INTENSITY OF EMOTION: check after each round

Set Up for Additional Tapping as needed

"Even though *I have some remaining* __________, I deeply and completely accept myself."

"This *remaining* _______.

NOTES: ________________________________

____

____

____

____

____

____

____

____

____

Date___________

<table>
<tr><td>

THE PROBLEM's "MOVIE TITLE"

</td></tr>
</table>

<table>
<tr><td>

THE NEGATIVE BELIEF/SELF-TALK:

</td></tr>
<tr><td>

Rate it: 1-100 (1= least intense, 100 = most intense)

</td></tr>
</table>

<table>
<tr><td colspan="2">

CONSIDER THE DETAILS (past/present/future):

</td></tr>
<tr><td>

WHAT event/condition happened?

WHO was/will be involved?

WHERE did/will it happen?

WHEN did/will it happen?

</td><td>

WHEN did it start?

WHAT was/is going on?

WHY did/will it happen?

HOW did/will it happen?

</td></tr>
<tr><td>

What does this REMIND me of?

What is the EARLIEST MEMORY this reminds me of?

</td><td>

What OTHER ISSUES came up?

What other SELF TALK attends this?

</td></tr>
</table>

<table>
<tr><td colspan="2">

What EMOTION & BODY SENSATIONS do I feel/notice?

</td></tr>
<tr><td>

Where is this felt?

Size? Shape? Edges?

</td><td>

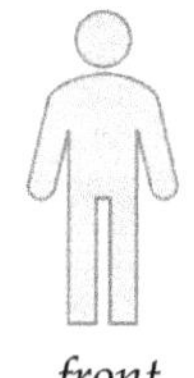 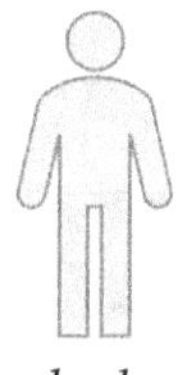

front   *back*

</td></tr>
<tr><td colspan="2">

Intensity of Emotion BEFORE tapping:

1 2 3 4 5 6 7 8 9 10   Low – Medium – High

</td></tr>
</table>

SET UP STATEMENT: 3x's at side of hand

"Even though

,*I deeply and completely accept myself"

Self-Acceptance Phrase

REMINDER PHRASE: at all other points

"This   in my

CHECK INTENSITY OF EMOTION: check after each round

Set Up for Additional Tapping as needed

"Even though *I have some remaining* __________, I deeply and completely accept myself."

"This *remaining* _______.

NOTES: ____

____

____

____

____

____

____

____

____

Date___________

<table>
<tr><td>

THE PROBLEM's "MOVIE TITLE"

</td></tr>
</table>

<table>
<tr><td>

THE NEGATIVE BELIEF/SELF-TALK:

</td></tr>
<tr><td>

Rate it: 1-100 (1= least intense, 100 = most intense)

</td></tr>
</table>

<table>
<tr><td colspan="2">

CONSIDER THE DETAILS (past/present/future):

</td></tr>
<tr><td>

WHAT event/condition happened?

WHO was/will be involved?

WHERE did/will it happen?

WHEN did/will it happen?

</td><td>

WHEN did it start?

WHAT was/is going on?

WHY did/will it happen?

HOW did/will it happen?

</td></tr>
<tr><td>

What does this REMIND me of?

What is the EARLIEST MEMORY this reminds me of?

</td><td>

What OTHER ISSUES came up?

What other SELF TALK attends this?

</td></tr>
</table>

<table>
<tr><td colspan="2">

What EMOTION & BODY SENSATIONS do I feel/notice?

</td></tr>
<tr><td>

Where is this felt?

Size? Shape? Edges?

</td><td>

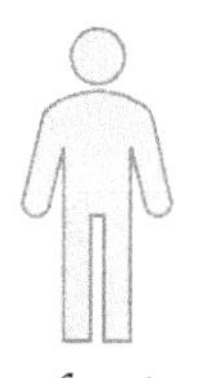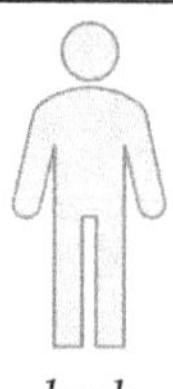

front   *back*

</td></tr>
<tr><td colspan="2">

Intensity of Emotion BEFORE tapping:

1 2 3 4 5 6 7 8 9 10   Low – Medium – High

</td></tr>
</table>

SET UP STATEMENT: 3x's at side of hand

> "Even though
>
>
>
>
>
> ,*I deeply and completely accept myself"

Self-Acceptance Phrase

REMINDER PHRASE: at all other points

> "This   in my

CHECK INTENSITY OF EMOTION: check after each round

Set Up for Additional Tapping as needed

"Even though *I have some remaining* _________, I deeply and completely accept myself."

"This *remaining* _______.

NOTES: ____

____

____

____

____

____

____

____

____

Date___________

<table>
<tr><td>

THE PROBLEM's "MOVIE TITLE"

</td></tr>
</table>

<table>
<tr><td>

THE NEGATIVE BELIEF/SELF-TALK:

</td></tr>
<tr><td>

Rate it: 1-100 (1= least intense, 100 = most intense)

</td></tr>
</table>

CONSIDER THE DETAILS (past/present/future):

WHAT event/condition happened?	WHEN did it start?
WHO was/will be involved?	WHAT was/is going on?
WHERE did/will it happen?	WHY did/will it happen?
WHEN did/will it happen?	HOW did/will it happen?

What does this REMIND me of?	What OTHER ISSUES came up?
What is the EARLIEST MEMORY this reminds me of?	What other SELF TALK attends this?

What EMOTION & BODY SENSATIONS do I feel/notice?

Where is this felt?

Size? Shape? Edges?

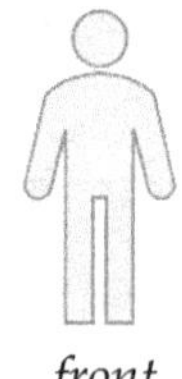 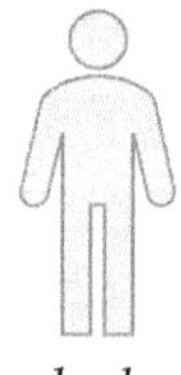

front　　　*back*

Intensity of Emotion BEFORE tapping:

1 2 3 4 5 6 7 8 9 10　　　Low – Medium – High

SET UP STATEMENT: 3x's at side of hand

"Even though

,*I deeply and completely accept myself"

Self-Acceptance Phrase

REMINDER PHRASE: at all other points

"This   in my

CHECK INTENSITY OF EMOTION: check after each round

Set Up for Additional Tapping as needed

"Even though ***I have some remaining*** ________, I deeply and completely accept myself."

"This ***remaining*** _______.

NOTES: _______________________________________

____

____

____

____

____

____

____

____

Date___________

THE PROBLEM's "MOVIE TITLE"

THE NEGATIVE BELIEF/SELF-TALK:

Rate it: 1-100 (1= least intense, 100 = most intense)

CONSIDER THE DETAILS (past/present/future):

WHAT event/condition happened?	WHEN did it start?
WHO was/will be involved?	WHAT was/is going on?
WHERE did/will it happen?	WHY did/will it happen?
WHEN did/will it happen?	HOW did/will it happen?

What does this REMIND me of?	What OTHER ISSUES came up?
What is the EARLIEST MEMORY this reminds me of?	What other SELF TALK attends this?

What EMOTION & BODY SENSATIONS do I feel/notice?

Where is this felt?

Size? Shape? Edges?

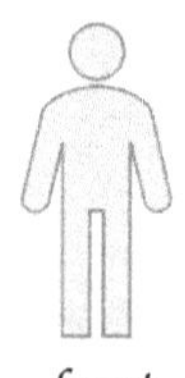 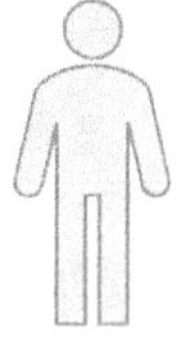

front   *back*

Intensity of Emotion BEFORE tapping:

1 2 3 4 5 6 7 8 9 10   Low – Medium – High

SET UP STATEMENT: 3x's at side of hand

"Even though

,*I deeply and completely accept myself"

Self-Acceptance Phrase

REMINDER PHRASE: at all other points

"This   in my

CHECK INTENSITY OF EMOTION: check after each round

Set Up for Additional Tapping as needed

"Even though *I have some remaining* _________, I deeply and completely accept myself."

"This *remaining* _______.

NOTES: ____

____

____

____

____

____

____

____

____

Date___________

<table>
<tr><td>

THE PROBLEM's "MOVIE TITLE"

</td></tr>
</table>

<table>
<tr><td>

THE NEGATIVE BELIEF/SELF-TALK:

Rate it: 1-100 (1= least intense, 100 = most intense)

</td></tr>
</table>

<table>
<tr><td colspan="2">

CONSIDER THE DETAILS (past/present/future):

</td></tr>
<tr><td>

WHAT event/condition happened?

WHO was/will be involved?

WHERE did/will it happen?

WHEN did/will it happen?

</td><td>

WHEN did it start?

WHAT was/is going on?

WHY did/will it happen?

HOW did/will it happen?

</td></tr>
<tr><td>

What does this REMIND me of?

What is the EARLIEST MEMORY this reminds me of?

</td><td>

What OTHER ISSUES came up?

What other SELF TALK attends this?

</td></tr>
</table>

<table>
<tr><td colspan="2">

What EMOTION & BODY SENSATIONS do I feel/notice?

</td></tr>
<tr><td>

Where is this felt?

Size? Shape? Edges?

</td><td>

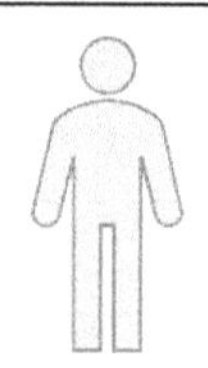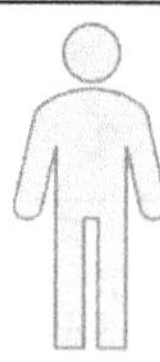

front   *back*

</td></tr>
</table>

Intensity of Emotion BEFORE tapping:

1 2 3 4 5 6 7 8 9 10   Low – Medium – High

SET UP STATEMENT: 3x's at side of hand

"Even though

,*I deeply and completely accept myself"

Self-Acceptance Phrase

REMINDER PHRASE: at all other points

"This   in my

CHECK INTENSITY OF EMOTION: check after each round

Set Up for Additional Tapping as needed

"Even though ***I have some remaining*** ________, I deeply and completely accept myself."

"This ***remaining*** ______.

NOTES: ____

____

____

____

____

____

____

____

Date___________

THE PROBLEM's "MOVIE TITLE"

THE NEGATIVE BELIEF/SELF-TALK:

Rate it: 1-100 (1= least intense, 100 = most intense)

CONSIDER THE DETAILS (past/present/future):

WHAT event/condition happened?	WHEN did it start?
WHO was/will be involved?	WHAT was/is going on?
WHERE did/will it happen?	WHY did/will it happen?
WHEN did/will it happen?	HOW did/will it happen?

What does this REMIND me of?	What OTHER ISSUES came up?
What is the EARLIEST MEMORY this reminds me of?	What other SELF TALK attends this?

What EMOTION & BODY SENSATIONS do I feel/notice?

Where is this felt?

Size? Shape? Edges?

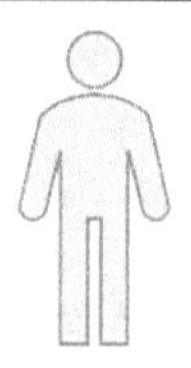
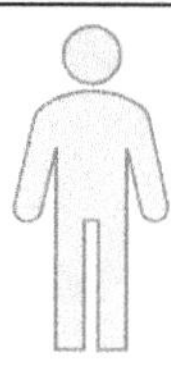

front *back*

Intensity of Emotion BEFORE tapping:

1 2 3 4 5 6 7 8 9 10   Low – Medium – High

SET UP STATEMENT: 3x's at side of hand

"Even though

,*I deeply and completely accept myself"

*Self-Acceptance Phrase

REMINDER PHRASE: at all other points

"This   in my

CHECK INTENSITY OF EMOTION: check after each round

Set Up for Additional Tapping as needed

"Even though *I have some remaining* __________, I deeply and completely accept myself."

"This *remaining* _______.

NOTES: ____

____

____

____

____

____

____

____

Date_______________

<table>
<tr><td>

THE PROBLEM's "MOVIE TITLE"

</td></tr>
</table>

<table>
<tr><td>

THE NEGATIVE BELIEF/SELF-TALK:

Rate it: 1-100 (1= least intense, 100 = most intense)

</td></tr>
</table>

CONSIDER THE DETAILS (past/present/future):

WHAT event/condition happened?	WHEN did it start?
WHO was/will be involved?	WHAT was/is going on?
WHERE did/will it happen?	WHY did/will it happen?
WHEN did/will it happen?	HOW did/will it happen?

What does this REMIND me of?	What OTHER ISSUES came up?
What is the EARLIEST MEMORY this reminds me of?	What other SELF TALK attends this?

What EMOTION & BODY SENSATIONS do I feel/notice?

Where is this felt?

Size? Shape? Edges?

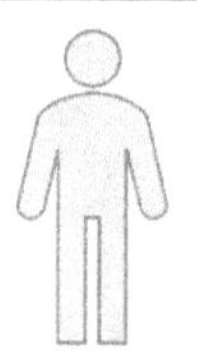 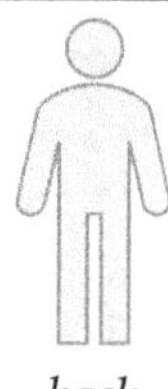

front   *back*

Intensity of Emotion BEFORE tapping:

1 2 3 4 5 6 7 8 9 10   Low – Medium – High

SET UP STATEMENT: 3x's at side of hand

"Even though

,*I deeply and completely accept myself"

Self-Acceptance Phrase

REMINDER PHRASE: at all other points

"This   in my

CHECK INTENSITY OF EMOTION: check after each round

Set Up for Additional Tapping as needed

"Even though *I have some remaining* __________, I deeply and completely accept myself."

"This *remaining* _______.

NOTES: ____

____

____

____

____

____

____

____

Date___________

<table>
<tr><td>

THE PROBLEM's "MOVIE TITLE"

</td></tr>
</table>

<table>
<tr><td>

THE NEGATIVE BELIEF/SELF-TALK:

</td></tr>
<tr><td>

Rate it: 1-100 (1= least intense, 100 = most intense)

</td></tr>
</table>

<table>
<tr><td colspan="2">

CONSIDER THE DETAILS (past/present/future):

</td></tr>
<tr><td>

WHAT event/condition happened?

WHO was/will be involved?

WHERE did/will it happen?

WHEN did/will it happen?

</td><td>

WHEN did it start?

WHAT was/is going on?

WHY did/will it happen?

HOW did/will it happen?

</td></tr>
<tr><td>

What does this REMIND me of?

What is the EARLIEST MEMORY this reminds me of?

</td><td>

What OTHER ISSUES came up?

What other SELF TALK attends this?

</td></tr>
</table>

<table>
<tr><td colspan="2">

What EMOTION & BODY SENSATIONS do I feel/notice?

</td></tr>
<tr><td>

Where is this felt?

Size? Shape? Edges?

</td><td>

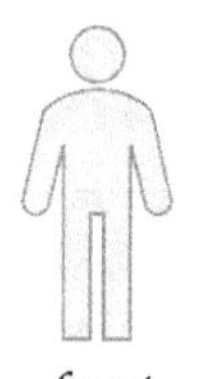 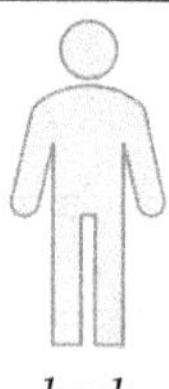

front   *back*

</td></tr>
<tr><td colspan="2">

Intensity of Emotion BEFORE tapping:

</td></tr>
<tr><td colspan="2">

1 2 3 4 5 6 7 8 9 10   Low – Medium – High

</td></tr>
</table>

SET UP STATEMENT: 3x's at side of hand

"Even though

,*I deeply and completely accept myself"

*Self-Acceptance Phrase

REMINDER PHRASE: at all other points

"This   in my

CHECK INTENSITY OF EMOTION: check after each round

Set Up for Additional Tapping as needed

"Even though *I have some remaining* _________, I deeply and completely accept myself."

"This *remaining* _______.

NOTES:

____

____

____

____

____

____

____

____

____

Date__________

<table>
<tr><td>THE PROBLEM's "MOVIE TITLE"</td></tr>
</table>

<table>
<tr><td>THE NEGATIVE BELIEF/SELF-TALK:</td></tr>
<tr><td>Rate it: 1-100 (1= least intense, 100 = most intense)</td></tr>
</table>

<table>
<tr><td colspan="2">CONSIDER THE DETAILS (past/present/future):</td></tr>
<tr>
<td>WHAT event/condition happened?
WHO was/will be involved?
WHERE did/will it happen?
WHEN did/will it happen?</td>
<td>WHEN did it start?
WHAT was/is going on?
WHY did/will it happen?
HOW did/will it happen?</td>
</tr>
<tr>
<td>What does this REMIND me of?
What is the EARLIEST MEMORY this reminds me of?</td>
<td>What OTHER ISSUES came up?
What other SELF TALK attends this?</td>
</tr>
</table>

<table>
<tr><td colspan="2">What EMOTION & BODY SENSATIONS do I feel/notice?</td></tr>
<tr>
<td>Where is this felt?
Size? Shape? Edges?</td>
<td>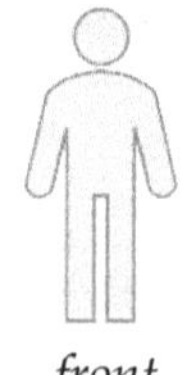 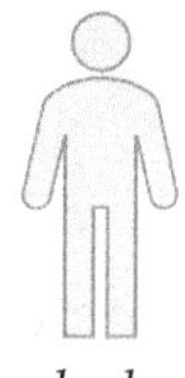
front   _back_</td>
</tr>
</table>

<table>
<tr><td colspan="2">Intensity of Emotion BEFORE tapping:</td></tr>
<tr><td>1 2 3 4 5 6 7 8 9 10</td><td>Low – Medium – High</td></tr>
</table>

SET UP STATEMENT: 3x's at side of hand

"Even though

,*I deeply and completely accept myself"

Self-Acceptance Phrase

REMINDER PHRASE: at all other points

"This   in my

CHECK INTENSITY OF EMOTION: check after each round

Set Up for Additional Tapping as needed

"Even though *I have some remaining* _________, I deeply and completely accept myself."

"This *remaining* _______.

NOTES: ____

____

____

____

____

____

____

____

____

Date___________

<table>
<tr><td>

THE PROBLEM's "MOVIE TITLE"

</td></tr>
</table>

<table>
<tr><td>

THE NEGATIVE BELIEF/SELF-TALK:

</td></tr>
<tr><td>

Rate it: 1-100 (1= least intense, 100 = most intense)

</td></tr>
</table>

<table>
<tr><td colspan="2">

CONSIDER THE DETAILS (past/present/future):

</td></tr>
<tr><td>

WHAT event/condition happened?

WHO was/will be involved?

WHERE did/will it happen?

WHEN did/will it happen?

</td><td>

WHEN did it start?

WHAT was/is going on?

WHY did/will it happen?

HOW did/will it happen?

</td></tr>
<tr><td>

What does this REMIND me of?

What is the EARLIEST MEMORY this reminds me of?

</td><td>

What OTHER ISSUES came up?

What other SELF TALK attends this?

</td></tr>
</table>

<table>
<tr><td colspan="2">

What EMOTION & BODY SENSATIONS do I feel/notice?

</td></tr>
<tr><td>

Where is this felt?

Size? Shape? Edges?

</td><td>

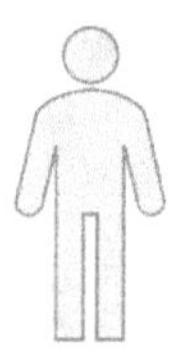 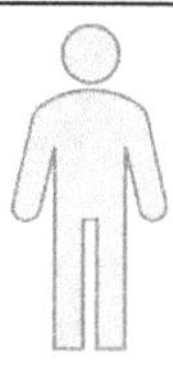

front   *back*

</td></tr>
<tr><td colspan="2">

Intensity of Emotion BEFORE tapping:

1 2 3 4 5 6 7 8 9 10   Low – Medium – High

</td></tr>
</table>

SET UP STATEMENT: 3x's at side of hand

"Even though

,*I deeply and completely accept myself"

Self-Acceptance Phrase

REMINDER PHRASE: at all other points

"This   in my

CHECK INTENSITY OF EMOTION: check after each round

Set Up for Additional Tapping as needed

"Even though *I have some remaining* _________, I deeply and completely accept myself."

"This *remaining* _______.

NOTES: ____

____

____

____

____

____

____

____

____

Date___________

THE PROBLEM's "MOVIE TITLE"

THE NEGATIVE BELIEF/SELF-TALK:

Rate it: 1-100 (1= least intense, 100 = most intense)

CONSIDER THE DETAILS (past/present/future):

WHAT event/condition happened?	WHEN did it start?
WHO was/will be involved?	WHAT was/is going on?
WHERE did/will it happen?	WHY did/will it happen?
WHEN did/will it happen?	HOW did/will it happen?

What does this REMIND me of?	What OTHER ISSUES came up?
What is the EARLIEST MEMORY this reminds me of?	What other SELF TALK attends this?

What EMOTION & BODY SENSATIONS do I feel/notice?

Where is this felt?

Size? Shape? Edges?

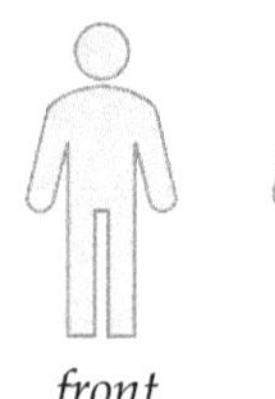 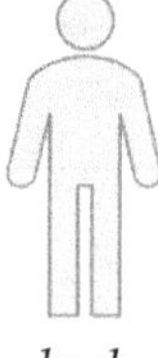

front   *back*

Intensity of Emotion BEFORE tapping:

1 2 3 4 5 6 7 8 9 10   Low – Medium – High

SET UP STATEMENT: 3x's at side of hand

"Even though

,*I deeply and completely accept myself"

Self-Acceptance Phrase

REMINDER PHRASE: at all other points

"This   in my

CHECK INTENSITY OF EMOTION: check after each round

Set Up for Additional Tapping as needed

"Even though *I have some remaining* _________, I deeply and completely accept myself."

"This *remaining* _______.

NOTES: ____

____

____

____

____

____

____

____

Date___________

<table>
<tr><td>

THE PROBLEM's "MOVIE TITLE"

</td></tr>
</table>

<table>
<tr><td>

THE NEGATIVE BELIEF/SELF-TALK:

</td></tr>
<tr><td>

Rate it: 1-100 (1= least intense, 100 = most intense)

</td></tr>
</table>

<table>
<tr><td colspan="2">

CONSIDER THE DETAILS (past/present/future):

</td></tr>
<tr><td>

WHAT event/condition happened?

WHO was/will be involved?

WHERE did/will it happen?

WHEN did/will it happen?

</td><td>

WHEN did it start?

WHAT was/is going on?

WHY did/will it happen?

HOW did/will it happen?

</td></tr>
<tr><td>

What does this REMIND me of?

What is the EARLIEST MEMORY this reminds me of?

</td><td>

What OTHER ISSUES came up?

What other SELF TALK attends this?

</td></tr>
</table>

<table>
<tr><td colspan="2">

What EMOTION & BODY SENSATIONS do I feel/notice?

</td></tr>
<tr><td>

Where is this felt?

Size? Shape? Edges?

</td><td>

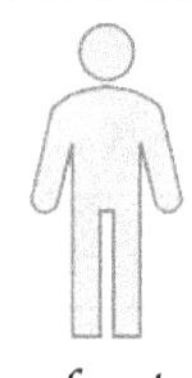 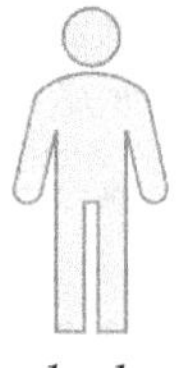

front   *back*

</td></tr>
<tr><td colspan="2">

Intensity of Emotion BEFORE tapping:

1 2 3 4 5 6 7 8 9 10   Low – Medium – High

</td></tr>
</table>

SET UP STATEMENT: 3x's at side of hand

> "Even though
>
>
>
>
>
> ,*I deeply and completely accept myself"

Self-Acceptance Phrase

REMINDER PHRASE: at all other points

> "This   in my

CHECK INTENSITY OF EMOTION: check after each round

Set Up for Additional Tapping as needed

"Even though *I have some remaining* __________, I deeply and completely accept myself."

"This *remaining* ______.

NOTES: ____

____

____

____

____

____

____

____

Date___________

THE PROBLEM's "MOVIE TITLE"

THE NEGATIVE BELIEF/SELF-TALK:

Rate it: 1-100 (1= least intense, 100 = most intense)

CONSIDER THE DETAILS (past/present/future):

WHAT event/condition happened?	WHEN did it start?
WHO was/will be involved?	WHAT was/is going on?
WHERE did/will it happen?	WHY did/will it happen?
WHEN did/will it happen?	HOW did/will it happen?

What does this REMIND me of?	What OTHER ISSUES came up?
What is the EARLIEST MEMORY this reminds me of?	What other SELF TALK attends this?

What EMOTION & BODY SENSATIONS do I feel/notice?

Where is this felt?

Size? Shape? Edges?

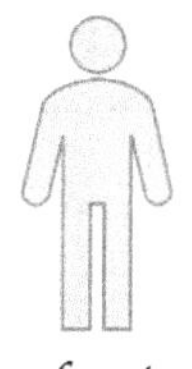 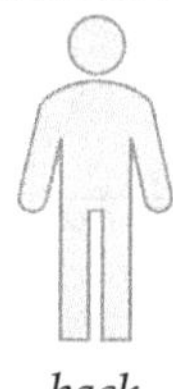

front   *back*

Intensity of Emotion BEFORE tapping:

1 2 3 4 5 6 7 8 9 10   Low – Medium – High

SET UP STATEMENT: 3x's at side of hand

"Even though

,*I deeply and completely accept myself"

Self-Acceptance Phrase

REMINDER PHRASE: at all other points

"This   in my

CHECK INTENSITY OF EMOTION: check after each round

Set Up for Additional Tapping as needed

"Even though *I have some remaining* __________, I deeply and completely accept myself."

"This *remaining* _______.

NOTES: ____

____

____

____

____

____

____

____

____

Date____________

<table>
<tr><td>

THE PROBLEM's "MOVIE TITLE"

</td></tr>
</table>

<table>
<tr><td>

THE NEGATIVE BELIEF/SELF-TALK:

</td></tr>
<tr><td>

Rate it: 1-100 (1= least intense, 100 = most intense)

</td></tr>
</table>

<table>
<tr><td colspan="2">

CONSIDER THE DETAILS (past/present/future):

</td></tr>
<tr><td>

WHAT event/condition happened?

WHO was/will be involved?

WHERE did/will it happen?

WHEN did/will it happen?

</td><td>

WHEN did it start?

WHAT was/is going on?

WHY did/will it happen?

HOW did/will it happen?

</td></tr>
<tr><td>

What does this REMIND me of?

What is the EARLIEST MEMORY this reminds me of?

</td><td>

What OTHER ISSUES came up?

What other SELF TALK attends this?

</td></tr>
</table>

<table>
<tr><td>

What EMOTION & BODY SENSATIONS do I feel/notice?

</td></tr>
<tr><td>

Where is this felt?

Size? Shape? Edges?

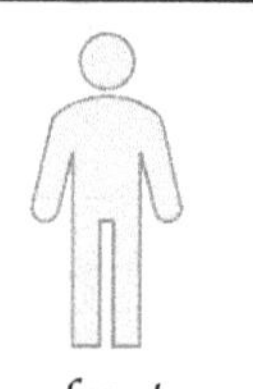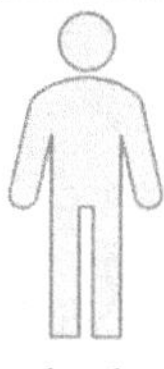

front   *back*

</td></tr>
<tr><td>

Intensity of Emotion BEFORE tapping:

1 2 3 4 5 6 7 8 9 10   Low – Medium – High

</td></tr>
</table>

SET UP STATEMENT: 3x's at side of hand

"Even though

,*I deeply and completely accept myself"

*Self-Acceptance Phrase

REMINDER PHRASE: at all other points

"This   in my

CHECK INTENSITY OF EMOTION: check after each round

Set Up for Additional Tapping as needed

"Even though *I have some remaining* ___________, I deeply and completely accept myself."

"This *remaining* _______.

NOTES: _______________________________________

____

____

____

____

____

____

____

____

____

Date___________

THE PROBLEM's "MOVIE TITLE"

THE NEGATIVE BELIEF/SELF-TALK:

Rate it: 1-100 (1= least intense, 100 = most intense)

CONSIDER THE DETAILS (past/present/future):

WHAT event/condition happened?	WHEN did it start?
WHO was/will be involved?	WHAT was/is going on?
WHERE did/will it happen?	WHY did/will it happen?
WHEN did/will it happen?	HOW did/will it happen?

What does this REMIND me of?	What OTHER ISSUES came up?
What is the EARLIEST MEMORY this reminds me of?	What other SELF TALK attends this?

What EMOTION & BODY SENSATIONS do I feel/notice?

Where is this felt?

Size? Shape? Edges?

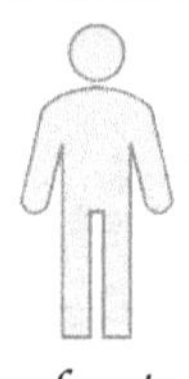 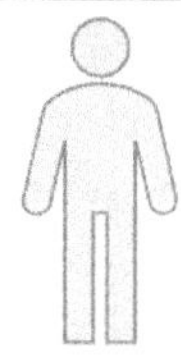

front   *back*

Intensity of Emotion BEFORE tapping:

1 2 3 4 5 6 7 8 9 10   Low – Medium – High

SET UP STATEMENT: 3x's at side of hand

> "Even though
>
>
>
>
> ,*I deeply and completely accept myself"

Self-Acceptance Phrase

REMINDER PHRASE: at all other points

"This   in my

CHECK INTENSITY OF EMOTION: check after each round

Set Up for Additional Tapping as needed

"Even though ***I have some remaining*** _________, I deeply and completely accept myself."

"This ***remaining*** _______.

NOTES: ____

____

____

____

____

____

____

____

____

Date___________

<table>
<tr><td>

THE PROBLEM's "MOVIE TITLE"

</td></tr>
</table>

<table>
<tr><td>

THE NEGATIVE BELIEF/SELF-TALK:

</td></tr>
<tr><td>

Rate it: 1-100 (1= least intense, 100 = most intense)

</td></tr>
</table>

CONSIDER THE DETAILS (past/present/future):

WHAT event/condition happened?	WHEN did it start?
WHO was/will be involved?	WHAT was/is going on?
WHERE did/will it happen?	WHY did/will it happen?
WHEN did/will it happen?	HOW did/will it happen?

What does this REMIND me of?	What OTHER ISSUES came up?
What is the EARLIEST MEMORY this reminds me of?	What other SELF TALK attends this?

What EMOTION & BODY SENSATIONS do I feel/notice?

Where is this felt?

Size? Shape? Edges?

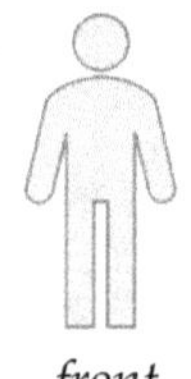 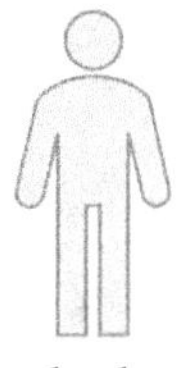

front   *back*

Intensity of Emotion BEFORE tapping:

1 2 3 4 5 6 7 8 9 10   Low – Medium – High

SET UP STATEMENT: 3x's at side of hand

"Even though

,*I deeply and completely accept myself"

Self-Acceptance Phrase

REMINDER PHRASE: at all other points

"This   in my

CHECK INTENSITY OF EMOTION: check after each round

Set Up for Additional Tapping as needed

"Even though ***I have some remaining*** _________, I deeply and completely accept myself."

"This ***remaining*** _______.

NOTES: ____

____

____

____

____

____

____

____

____

Date____________

<table>
<tr><td>

THE PROBLEM's "MOVIE TITLE"

</td></tr>
</table>

<table>
<tr><td>

THE NEGATIVE BELIEF/SELF-TALK:

Rate it: 1-100 (1= least intense, 100 = most intense)

</td></tr>
</table>

<table>
<tr><td>

CONSIDER THE DETAILS (past/present/future):

WHAT event/condition happened?	WHEN did it start?
WHO was/will be involved?	WHAT was/is going on?
WHERE did/will it happen?	WHY did/will it happen?
WHEN did/will it happen?	HOW did/will it happen?

What does this REMIND me of?	What OTHER ISSUES came up?
What is the EARLIEST MEMORY this reminds me of?	What other SELF TALK attends this?

</td></tr>
</table>

<table>
<tr><td>

What EMOTION & BODY SENSATIONS do I feel/notice?

Where is this felt?

Size? Shape? Edges?

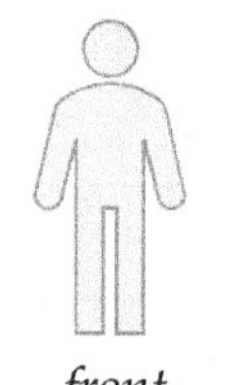 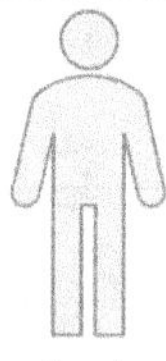

front   *back*

Intensity of Emotion BEFORE tapping:

1 2 3 4 5 6 7 8 9 10   Low – Medium – High

</td></tr>
</table>

SET UP STATEMENT: 3x's at side of hand

"Even though

,*I deeply and completely accept myself"

*Self-Acceptance Phrase

REMINDER PHRASE: at all other points

"This   in my

CHECK INTENSITY OF EMOTION: check after each round

Set Up for Additional Tapping as needed

"Even though *I have some remaining* _________, I deeply and completely accept myself."

"This *remaining* _______.

NOTES: ____

____

____

____

____

____

____

____

____

Date___________

<table>
<tr><td>

THE PROBLEM's "MOVIE TITLE"

</td></tr>
</table>

<table>
<tr><td>

THE NEGATIVE BELIEF/SELF-TALK:

Rate it: 1-100 (1= least intense, 100 = most intense)

</td></tr>
</table>

<table>
<tr><td colspan="2">

CONSIDER THE DETAILS (past/present/future):

</td></tr>
<tr><td>

WHAT event/condition happened?

WHO was/will be involved?

WHERE did/will it happen?

WHEN did/will it happen?

</td><td>

WHEN did it start?

WHAT was/is going on?

WHY did/will it happen?

HOW did/will it happen?

</td></tr>
<tr><td>

What does this REMIND me of?

What is the EARLIEST MEMORY this reminds me of?

</td><td>

What OTHER ISSUES came up?

What other SELF TALK attends this?

</td></tr>
</table>

<table>
<tr><td colspan="2">

What EMOTION & BODY SENSATIONS do I feel/notice?

</td></tr>
<tr><td>

Where is this felt?

Size? Shape? Edges?

</td><td>

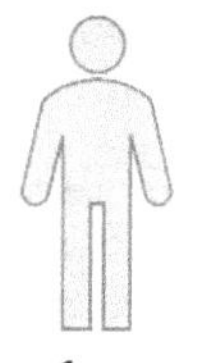 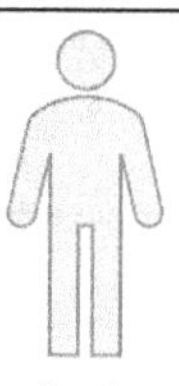

front   *back*

</td></tr>
<tr><td colspan="2">

Intensity of Emotion BEFORE tapping:

1 2 3 4 5 6 7 8 9 10   Low – Medium – High

</td></tr>
</table>

SET UP STATEMENT: 3x's at side of hand

"Even though

,*I deeply and completely accept myself"

Self-Acceptance Phrase

REMINDER PHRASE: at all other points

"This   in my

CHECK INTENSITY OF EMOTION: check after each round

Set Up for Additional Tapping as needed

"Even though *I have some remaining* ________, I deeply and completely accept myself."

"This *remaining* ______.

NOTES: ______________________________________

____

____

____

____

____

____

____

Date___________

THE PROBLEM's "MOVIE TITLE"

THE NEGATIVE BELIEF/SELF-TALK:
Rate it: 1-100 (1= least intense, 100 = most intense)

CONSIDER THE DETAILS (past/present/future):

WHAT event/condition happened?	WHEN did it start?
WHO was/will be involved?	WHAT was/is going on?
WHERE did/will it happen?	WHY did/will it happen?
WHEN did/will it happen?	HOW did/will it happen?

What does this REMIND me of?	What OTHER ISSUES came up?
What is the EARLIEST MEMORY this reminds me of?	What other SELF TALK attends this?

What EMOTION & BODY SENSATIONS do I feel/notice?

Where is this felt?

Size? Shape? Edges?

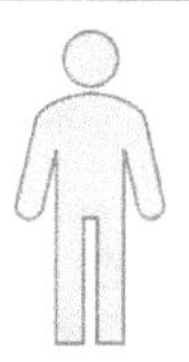
front

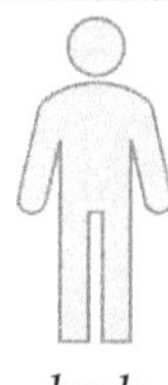
back

Intensity of Emotion BEFORE tapping:

1 2 3 4 5 6 7 8 9 10   Low – Medium – High

SET UP STATEMENT: 3x's at side of hand

"Even though

,*I deeply and completely accept myself"

Self-Acceptance Phrase

REMINDER PHRASE: at all other points

"This   in my

CHECK INTENSITY OF EMOTION: check after each round

Set Up for Additional Tapping as needed

"Even though **I have some remaining** _________, I deeply and completely accept myself."

"This **remaining** _______.

NOTES: _______________________________________

____

____

____

____

____

____

____

____

Date_____________

<table>
<tr><td>

THE PROBLEM's "MOVIE TITLE"

</td></tr>
</table>

<table>
<tr><td>

THE NEGATIVE BELIEF/SELF-TALK:

</td></tr>
<tr><td>

Rate it: 1-100 (1= least intense, 100 = most intense)

</td></tr>
</table>

<table>
<tr><td colspan="2">

CONSIDER THE DETAILS (past/present/future):

</td></tr>
<tr><td>

WHAT event/condition happened?

WHO was/will be involved?

WHERE did/will it happen?

WHEN did/will it happen?

</td><td>

WHEN did it start?

WHAT was/is going on?

WHY did/will it happen?

HOW did/will it happen?

</td></tr>
<tr><td>

What does this REMIND me of?

What is the EARLIEST MEMORY this reminds me of?

</td><td>

What OTHER ISSUES came up?

What other SELF TALK attends this?

</td></tr>
</table>

<table>
<tr><td colspan="2">

What EMOTION & BODY SENSATIONS do I feel/notice?

</td></tr>
<tr><td>

Where is this felt?

Size? Shape? Edges?

</td><td>

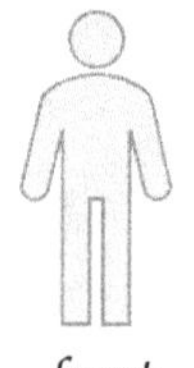 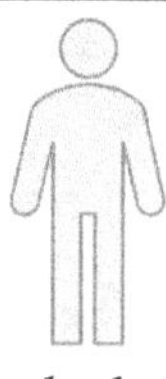

front   *back*

</td></tr>
<tr><td colspan="2">

Intensity of Emotion BEFORE tapping:

</td></tr>
<tr><td colspan="2">

1 2 3 4 5 6 7 8 9 10   Low – Medium – High

</td></tr>
</table>

SET UP STATEMENT: 3x's at side of hand

"Even though

,*I deeply and completely accept myself"

Self-Acceptance Phrase

REMINDER PHRASE: at all other points

"This   in my

CHECK INTENSITY OF EMOTION: check after each round

Set Up for Additional Tapping as needed

"Even though *I have some remaining* _________, I deeply and completely accept myself."

"This *remaining* _______.

NOTES: ____

____

____

____

____

____

____

____

____

Date___________

<table>
<tr><td>

THE PROBLEM's "MOVIE TITLE"

</td></tr>
</table>

<table>
<tr><td>

THE NEGATIVE BELIEF/SELF-TALK:

</td></tr>
<tr><td>

Rate it: 1-100 (1= least intense, 100 = most intense)

</td></tr>
</table>

<table>
<tr><td colspan="2">

CONSIDER THE DETAILS (past/present/future):

</td></tr>
<tr><td>

WHAT event/condition happened?

WHO was/will be involved?

WHERE did/will it happen?

WHEN did/will it happen?

</td><td>

WHEN did it start?

WHAT was/is going on?

WHY did/will it happen?

HOW did/will it happen?

</td></tr>
<tr><td>

What does this REMIND me of?

What is the EARLIEST MEMORY this reminds me of?

</td><td>

What OTHER ISSUES came up?

What other SELF TALK attends this?

</td></tr>
</table>

<table>
<tr><td colspan="2">

What EMOTION & BODY SENSATIONS do I feel/notice?

</td></tr>
<tr><td>

Where is this felt?

Size? Shape? Edges?

</td><td>

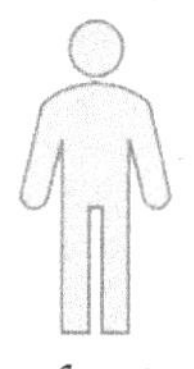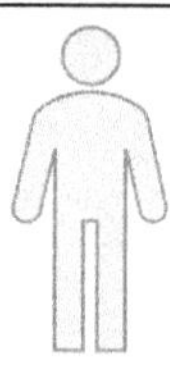

front   *back*

</td></tr>
<tr><td colspan="2">

Intensity of Emotion BEFORE tapping:

</td></tr>
<tr><td colspan="2">

1 2 3 4 5 6 7 8 9 10   Low – Medium – High

</td></tr>
</table>

SET UP STATEMENT: 3x's at side of hand

> "Even though
>
>
>
>
>
> ,*I deeply and completely accept myself"

Self-Acceptance Phrase

REMINDER PHRASE: at all other points

"This   in my

CHECK INTENSITY OF EMOTION: check after each round

Set Up for Additional Tapping as needed

"Even though **I have some remaining** _________, I deeply and completely accept myself."

"This **remaining** _______.

NOTES: ___________________________________

____

____

____

____

____

____

____

____

Date________________

<table>
<tr><td>

THE PROBLEM's "MOVIE TITLE"

</td></tr>
</table>

<table>
<tr><td>

THE NEGATIVE BELIEF/SELF-TALK:

</td></tr>
<tr><td>

Rate it: 1-100 (1= least intense, 100 = most intense)

</td></tr>
</table>

<table>
<tr><td colspan="2">

CONSIDER THE DETAILS (past/present/future):

</td></tr>
<tr><td>

WHAT event/condition happened?

WHO was/will be involved?

WHERE did/will it happen?

WHEN did/will it happen?

</td><td>

WHEN did it start?

WHAT was/is going on?

WHY did/will it happen?

HOW did/will it happen?

</td></tr>
<tr><td>

What does this REMIND me of?

What is the EARLIEST MEMORY this reminds me of?

</td><td>

What OTHER ISSUES came up?

What other SELF TALK attends this?

</td></tr>
</table>

<table>
<tr><td colspan="2">

What EMOTION & BODY SENSATIONS do I feel/notice?

</td></tr>
<tr><td>

Where is this felt?

Size? Shape? Edges?

</td><td>

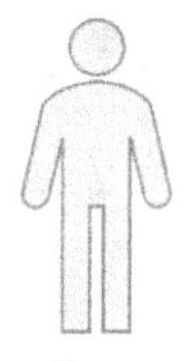 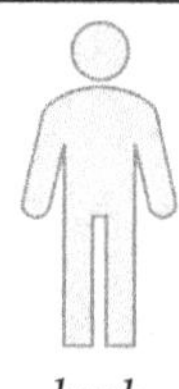

front　　*back*

</td></tr>
<tr><td colspan="2">

Intensity of Emotion BEFORE tapping:

1 2 3 4 5 6 7 8 9 10　　　　　Low – Medium – High

</td></tr>
</table>

SET UP STATEMENT: 3x's at side of hand

"Even though

,*I deeply and completely accept myself"

Self-Acceptance Phrase

REMINDER PHRASE: at all other points

"This   in my

CHECK INTENSITY OF EMOTION: check after each round

Set Up for Additional Tapping as needed

"Even though *I have some remaining* _________, I deeply and completely accept myself."

"This *remaining* _______.

NOTES: ____

____

____

____

____

____

____

____

____

Date____________

THE PROBLEM's "MOVIE TITLE"

THE NEGATIVE BELIEF/SELF-TALK:

Rate it: 1-100 (1= least intense, 100 = most intense)

CONSIDER THE DETAILS (past/present/future):

WHAT event/condition happened?	WHEN did it start?
WHO was/will be involved?	WHAT was/is going on?
WHERE did/will it happen?	WHY did/will it happen?
WHEN did/will it happen?	HOW did/will it happen?

What does this REMIND me of?	What OTHER ISSUES came up?
What is the EARLIEST MEMORY this reminds me of?	What other SELF TALK attends this?

What EMOTION & BODY SENSATIONS do I feel/notice?

Where is this felt?

Size? Shape? Edges?

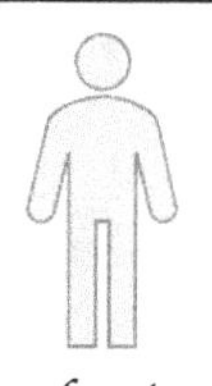 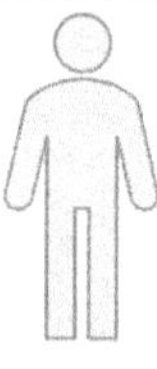

front   *back*

Intensity of Emotion BEFORE tapping:

1 2 3 4 5 6 7 8 9 10   Low – Medium – High

SET UP STATEMENT: 3x's at side of hand

"Even though

,*I deeply and completely accept myself"

Self-Acceptance Phrase

REMINDER PHRASE: at all other points

"This   in my

CHECK INTENSITY OF EMOTION: check after each round

Set Up for Additional Tapping as needed

"Even though *I have some remaining* _________, I deeply and completely accept myself."

"This *remaining* _______.

NOTES: _______________________________________

____

____

____

____

____

____

____

____

Date___________

THE PROBLEM's "MOVIE TITLE"

THE NEGATIVE BELIEF/SELF-TALK:

Rate it: 1-100 (1= least intense, 100 = most intense)

CONSIDER THE DETAILS (past/present/future):

WHAT event/condition happened?	WHEN did it start?
WHO was/will be involved?	WHAT was/is going on?
WHERE did/will it happen?	WHY did/will it happen?
WHEN did/will it happen?	HOW did/will it happen?

What does this REMIND me of?	What OTHER ISSUES came up?
What is the EARLIEST MEMORY this reminds me of?	What other SELF TALK attends this?

What EMOTION & BODY SENSATIONS do I feel/notice?

Where is this felt?

Size? Shape? Edges?

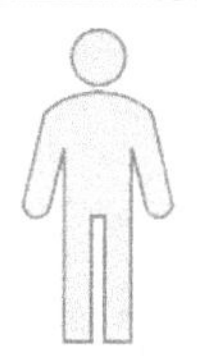 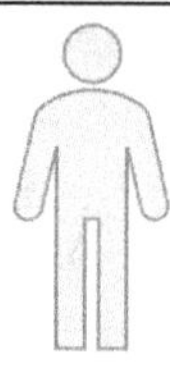

Intensity of Emotion BEFORE tapping:

1 2 3 4 5 6 7 8 9 10   Low – Medium – High

SET UP STATEMENT: 3x's at side of hand

"Even though

,*I deeply and completely accept myself"

Self-Acceptance Phrase

REMINDER PHRASE: at all other points

"This   in my

CHECK INTENSITY OF EMOTION: check after each round

Set Up for Additional Tapping as needed

"Even though *I have some remaining* __________, I deeply and completely accept myself."

"This *remaining* _______.

NOTES: _______________________________________

____

____

____

____

____

____

____

____

Date____________

<table>
<tr><td>

THE PROBLEM's "MOVIE TITLE"

</td></tr>
</table>

<table>
<tr><td>

THE NEGATIVE BELIEF/SELF-TALK:

</td></tr>
<tr><td>

Rate it: 1-100 (1= least intense, 100 = most intense)

</td></tr>
</table>

<table>
<tr><td colspan="2">

CONSIDER THE DETAILS (past/present/future):

</td></tr>
<tr><td>

WHAT event/condition happened?

WHO was/will be involved?

WHERE did/will it happen?

WHEN did/will it happen?

</td><td>

WHEN did it start?

WHAT was/is going on?

WHY did/will it happen?

HOW did/will it happen?

</td></tr>
<tr><td>

What does this REMIND me of?

What is the EARLIEST MEMORY this reminds me of?

</td><td>

What OTHER ISSUES came up?

What other SELF TALK attends this?

</td></tr>
</table>

<table>
<tr><td colspan="2">

What EMOTION & BODY SENSATIONS do I feel/notice?

</td></tr>
<tr><td>

Where is this felt?

Size? Shape? Edges?

</td><td>

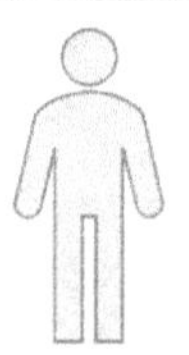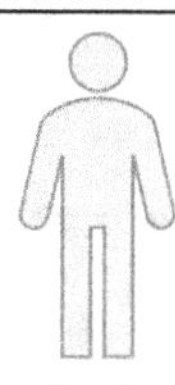

front   *back*

</td></tr>
<tr><td colspan="2">

Intensity of Emotion BEFORE tapping:

</td></tr>
<tr><td colspan="2">

1 2 3 4 5 6 7 8 9 10   Low – Medium – High

</td></tr>
</table>

SET UP STATEMENT: 3x's at side of hand

"Even though

,*I deeply and completely accept myself"

Self-Acceptance Phrase

REMINDER PHRASE: at all other points

"This   in my

CHECK INTENSITY OF EMOTION: check after each round

Set Up for Additional Tapping as needed

"Even though ***I have some remaining*** _________, I deeply and completely accept myself."

"This ***remaining*** _______.

NOTES: _______________________________________

____

____

____

____

____

____

____

Date___________

THE PROBLEM's "MOVIE TITLE"

THE NEGATIVE BELIEF/SELF-TALK:

Rate it: 1-100 (1= least intense, 100 = most intense)

CONSIDER THE DETAILS (past/present/future):

WHAT event/condition happened?	WHEN did it start?
WHO was/will be involved?	WHAT was/is going on?
WHERE did/will it happen?	WHY did/will it happen?
WHEN did/will it happen?	HOW did/will it happen?

What does this REMIND me of?	What OTHER ISSUES came up?
What is the EARLIEST MEMORY this reminds me of?	What other SELF TALK attends this?

What EMOTION & BODY SENSATIONS do I feel/notice?

Where is this felt?

Size? Shape? Edges?

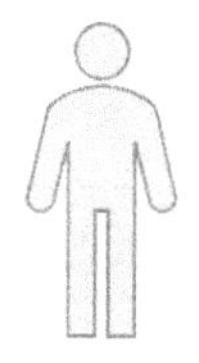 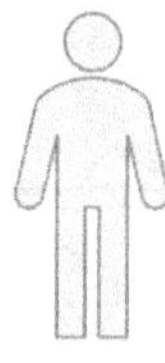

front   *back*

Intensity of Emotion BEFORE tapping:

1 2 3 4 5 6 7 8 9 10   Low – Medium – High

SET UP STATEMENT: 3x's at side of hand

"Even though

,*I deeply and completely accept myself"

Self-Acceptance Phrase

REMINDER PHRASE: at all other points

"This   in my

CHECK INTENSITY OF EMOTION: check after each round

Set Up for Additional Tapping as needed

"Even though *I have some remaining* __________, I deeply and completely accept myself."

"This *remaining* ________.

NOTES: _______________________________________

____

____

____

____

____

____

____

____

Date___________

THE PROBLEM's "MOVIE TITLE"

THE NEGATIVE BELIEF/SELF-TALK:

Rate it: 1-100 (1= least intense, 100 = most intense)

CONSIDER THE DETAILS (past/present/future):

WHAT event/condition happened?	WHEN did it start?
WHO was/will be involved?	WHAT was/is going on?
WHERE did/will it happen?	WHY did/will it happen?
WHEN did/will it happen?	HOW did/will it happen?

What does this REMIND me of?	What OTHER ISSUES came up?
What is the EARLIEST MEMORY this reminds me of?	What other SELF TALK attends this?

What EMOTION & BODY SENSATIONS do I feel/notice?

Where is this felt?

Size? Shape? Edges?

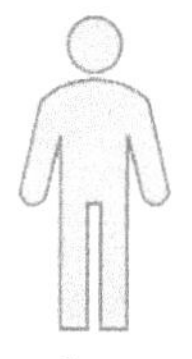

front

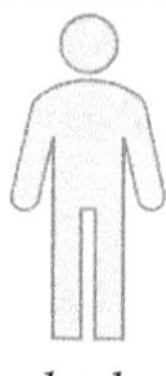

back

Intensity of Emotion BEFORE tapping:

1 2 3 4 5 6 7 8 9 10   Low – Medium – High

SET UP STATEMENT: 3x's at side of hand

"Even though

,*I deeply and completely accept myself"

*Self-Acceptance Phrase

REMINDER PHRASE: at all other points

"This   in my

CHECK INTENSITY OF EMOTION: check after each round

Set Up for Additional Tapping as needed

"Even though *I have some remaining* _________, I deeply and completely accept myself."

"This *remaining* _______.

NOTES: ____

____

____

____

____

____

____

____

____

Date___________

<table>
<tr><td>

THE PROBLEM's "MOVIE TITLE"

</td></tr>
</table>

<table>
<tr><td>

THE NEGATIVE BELIEF/SELF-TALK:

</td></tr>
<tr><td>

Rate it: 1-100 (1= least intense, 100 = most intense)

</td></tr>
</table>

<table>
<tr><td colspan="2">

CONSIDER THE DETAILS (past/present/future):

</td></tr>
<tr><td>

WHAT event/condition happened?

WHO was/will be involved?

WHERE did/will it happen?

WHEN did/will it happen?

</td><td>

WHEN did it start?

WHAT was/is going on?

WHY did/will it happen?

HOW did/will it happen?

</td></tr>
<tr><td>

What does this REMIND me of?

What is the EARLIEST MEMORY this reminds me of?

</td><td>

What OTHER ISSUES came up?

What other SELF TALK attends this?

</td></tr>
</table>

<table>
<tr><td colspan="2">

What EMOTION & BODY SENSATIONS do I feel/notice?

</td></tr>
<tr><td>

Where is this felt?

Size? Shape? Edges?

</td><td>

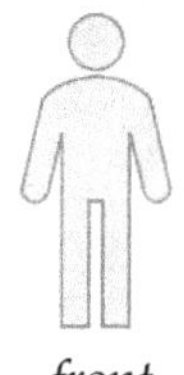 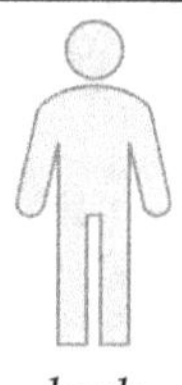

front　　　*back*

</td></tr>
</table>

<table>
<tr><td>

Intensity of Emotion BEFORE tapping:

</td></tr>
<tr><td>

1 2 3 4 5 6 7 8 9 10　　　　　Low – Medium – High

</td></tr>
</table>

SET UP STATEMENT: 3x's at side of hand

"Even though

,*I deeply and completely accept myself"

Self-Acceptance Phrase

REMINDER PHRASE: at all other points

"This   in my

CHECK INTENSITY OF EMOTION: check after each round

Set Up for Additional Tapping as needed

"Even though **I have some remaining** _________, I deeply and completely accept myself."

"This **remaining** _______.

NOTES: ____

____

____

____

____

____

____

____

____

Date____________

<table>
<tr><td>

THE PROBLEM's "MOVIE TITLE"

</td></tr>
</table>

<table>
<tr><td>

THE NEGATIVE BELIEF/SELF-TALK:

</td></tr>
<tr><td>

Rate it: 1-100 (1= least intense, 100 = most intense)

</td></tr>
</table>

<table>
<tr><td colspan="2">

CONSIDER THE DETAILS (past/present/future):

</td></tr>
<tr><td>

WHAT event/condition happened?

WHO was/will be involved?

WHERE did/will it happen?

WHEN did/will it happen?

</td><td>

WHEN did it start?

WHAT was/is going on?

WHY did/will it happen?

HOW did/will it happen?

</td></tr>
<tr><td>

What does this REMIND me of?

What is the EARLIEST MEMORY this reminds me of?

</td><td>

What OTHER ISSUES came up?

What other SELF TALK attends this?

</td></tr>
</table>

<table>
<tr><td colspan="2">

What EMOTION & BODY SENSATIONS do I feel/notice?

</td></tr>
<tr><td>

Where is this felt?

Size? Shape? Edges?

</td><td>

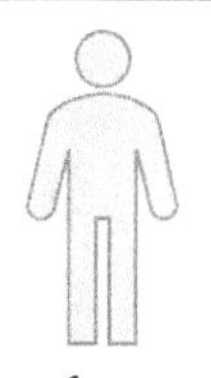 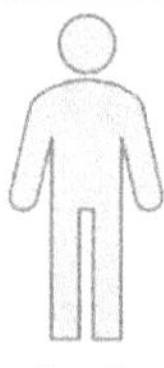

front   *back*

</td></tr>
<tr><td colspan="2">

Intensity of Emotion BEFORE tapping:

</td></tr>
<tr><td colspan="2">

1 2 3 4 5 6 7 8 9 10   Low – Medium – High

</td></tr>
</table>

SET UP STATEMENT: 3x's at side of hand

"Even though

,*I deeply and completely accept myself"

*Self-Acceptance Phrase

REMINDER PHRASE: at all other points

"This   in my

CHECK INTENSITY OF EMOTION: check after each round

Set Up for Additional Tapping as needed

"Even though *I have some remaining* __________, I deeply and completely accept myself."

"This *remaining* ________.

NOTES: ____

____

____

____

____

____

____

____

____

Date___________

<table>
<tr><td>

THE PROBLEM's "MOVIE TITLE"

</td></tr>
</table>

<table>
<tr><td>

THE NEGATIVE BELIEF/SELF-TALK:

</td></tr>
<tr><td>

Rate it: 1-100 (1= least intense, 100 = most intense)

</td></tr>
</table>

<table>
<tr><td colspan="2">

CONSIDER THE DETAILS (past/present/future):

</td></tr>
<tr><td>

WHAT event/condition happened?

WHO was/will be involved?

WHERE did/will it happen?

WHEN did/will it happen?

</td><td>

WHEN did it start?

WHAT was/is going on?

WHY did/will it happen?

HOW did/will it happen?

</td></tr>
<tr><td>

What does this REMIND me of?

What is the EARLIEST MEMORY this reminds me of?

</td><td>

What OTHER ISSUES came up?

What other SELF TALK attends this?

</td></tr>
</table>

<table>
<tr><td colspan="2">

What EMOTION & BODY SENSATIONS do I feel/notice?

</td></tr>
<tr><td>

Where is this felt?

Size? Shape? Edges?

</td><td>

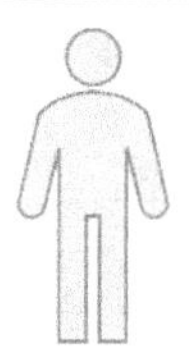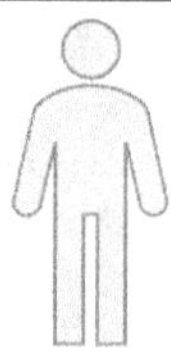

front   *back*

</td></tr>
</table>

<table>
<tr><td colspan="2">

Intensity of Emotion BEFORE tapping:

</td></tr>
<tr><td>

1 2 3 4 5 6 7 8 9 10

</td><td>

Low – Medium – High

</td></tr>
</table>

SET UP STATEMENT: 3x's at side of hand

"Even though

,*I deeply and completely accept myself"

*Self-Acceptance Phrase

REMINDER PHRASE: at all other points

"This   in my

CHECK INTENSITY OF EMOTION: check after each round

Set Up for Additional Tapping as needed

"Even though *I have some remaining* _________, I deeply and completely accept myself."

"This *remaining* _______.

NOTES: ____

____

____

____

____

____

____

____

____

Date___________

<table>
<tr><td>

THE PROBLEM's "MOVIE TITLE"

</td></tr>
</table>

<table>
<tr><td>

THE NEGATIVE BELIEF/SELF-TALK:

</td></tr>
<tr><td>

Rate it: 1-100 (1= least intense, 100 = most intense)

</td></tr>
</table>

<table>
<tr><td colspan="2">

CONSIDER THE DETAILS (past/present/future):

</td></tr>
<tr><td>

WHAT event/condition happened?

WHO was/will be involved?

WHERE did/will it happen?

WHEN did/will it happen?

</td><td>

WHEN did it start?

WHAT was/is going on?

WHY did/will it happen?

HOW did/will it happen?

</td></tr>
<tr><td>

What does this REMIND me of?

What is the EARLIEST MEMORY this reminds me of?

</td><td>

What OTHER ISSUES came up?

What other SELF TALK attends this?

</td></tr>
</table>

<table>
<tr><td colspan="2">

What EMOTION & BODY SENSATIONS do I feel/notice?

</td></tr>
<tr><td>

Where is this felt?

Size? Shape? Edges?

</td><td>

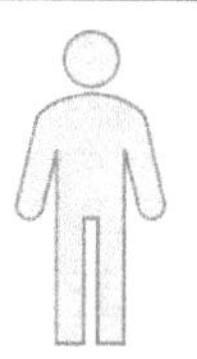 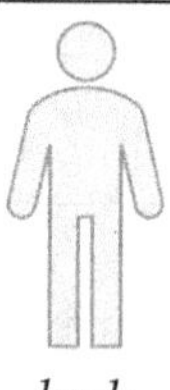

front   *back*

</td></tr>
<tr><td colspan="2">

Intensity of Emotion BEFORE tapping:

</td></tr>
<tr><td colspan="2">

1 2 3 4 5 6 7 8 9 10   Low – Medium – High

</td></tr>
</table>

SET UP STATEMENT: 3x's at side of hand

"Even though

,*I deeply and completely accept myself"

Self-Acceptance Phrase

REMINDER PHRASE: at all other points

"This   in my

CHECK INTENSITY OF EMOTION: check after each round

Set Up for Additional Tapping as needed

"Even though **I have some remaining** __________, I deeply and completely accept myself."

"This **remaining** _______.

NOTES: _______________________________________

____

____

____

____

____

____

____

Date___________

<table>
<tr><td>

THE PROBLEM's "MOVIE TITLE"

</td></tr>
</table>

<table>
<tr><td>

THE NEGATIVE BELIEF/SELF-TALK:

Rate it: 1-100 (1= least intense, 100 = most intense)

</td></tr>
</table>

<table>
<tr><td colspan="2">

CONSIDER THE DETAILS (past/present/future):

</td></tr>
<tr><td>

WHAT event/condition happened?

WHO was/will be involved?

WHERE did/will it happen?

WHEN did/will it happen?

</td><td>

WHEN did it start?

WHAT was/is going on?

WHY did/will it happen?

HOW did/will it happen?

</td></tr>
<tr><td>

What does this REMIND me of?

What is the EARLIEST MEMORY this reminds me of?

</td><td>

What OTHER ISSUES came up?

What other SELF TALK attends this?

</td></tr>
</table>

<table>
<tr><td colspan="2">

What EMOTION & BODY SENSATIONS do I feel/notice?

</td></tr>
<tr><td>

Where is this felt?

Size? Shape? Edges?

</td><td>

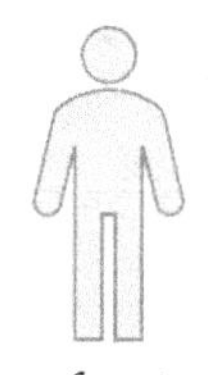 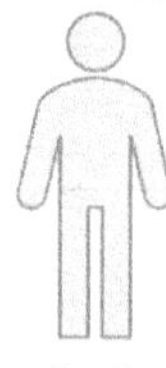

front   *back*

</td></tr>
</table>

Intensity of Emotion BEFORE tapping:

1 2 3 4 5 6 7 8 9 10   Low – Medium – High

SET UP STATEMENT: 3x's at side of hand

"Even though

,*I deeply and completely accept myself"

Self-Acceptance Phrase

REMINDER PHRASE: at all other points

"This   in my

CHECK INTENSITY OF EMOTION: check after each round

Set Up for Additional Tapping as needed

"Even though *I have some remaining* _________, I deeply and completely accept myself."

"This *remaining* _______.

NOTES: ____

____

____

____

____

____

____

____

____

Date___________

THE PROBLEM's "MOVIE TITLE"

THE NEGATIVE BELIEF/SELF-TALK:

Rate it: 1-100 (1= least intense, 100 = most intense)

CONSIDER THE DETAILS (past/present/future):

WHAT event/condition happened?	WHEN did it start?
WHO was/will be involved?	WHAT was/is going on?
WHERE did/will it happen?	WHY did/will it happen?
WHEN did/will it happen?	HOW did/will it happen?

What does this REMIND me of?	What OTHER ISSUES came up?
What is the EARLIEST MEMORY this reminds me of?	What other SELF TALK attends this?

What EMOTION & BODY SENSATIONS do I feel/notice?

Where is this felt?

Size? Shape? Edges?

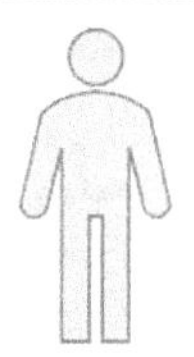 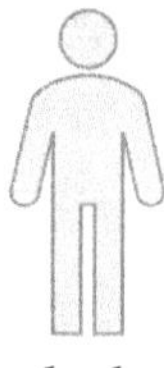

front   *back*

Intensity of Emotion BEFORE tapping:

1 2 3 4 5 6 7 8 9 10   Low – Medium – High

SET UP STATEMENT: 3x's at side of hand

"Even though

,*I deeply and completely accept myself"

*Self-Acceptance Phrase

REMINDER PHRASE: at all other points

"This   in my

CHECK INTENSITY OF EMOTION: check after each round

Set Up for Additional Tapping as needed

"Even though *I have some remaining* ________, I deeply and completely accept myself."

"This *remaining* _______.

NOTES: ____

____

____

____

____

____

____

____

Date___________

<table>
<tr><td>

THE PROBLEM's "MOVIE TITLE"

</td></tr>
</table>

<table>
<tr><td>

THE NEGATIVE BELIEF/SELF-TALK:

</td></tr>
<tr><td>

Rate it: 1-100 (1= least intense, 100 = most intense)

</td></tr>
</table>

<table>
<tr><td colspan="2">

CONSIDER THE DETAILS (past/present/future):

</td></tr>
<tr><td>

WHAT event/condition happened?

WHO was/will be involved?

WHERE did/will it happen?

WHEN did/will it happen?

</td><td>

WHEN did it start?

WHAT was/is going on?

WHY did/will it happen?

HOW did/will it happen?

</td></tr>
<tr><td>

What does this REMIND me of?

What is the EARLIEST MEMORY this reminds me of?

</td><td>

What OTHER ISSUES came up?

What other SELF TALK attends this?

</td></tr>
</table>

<table>
<tr><td colspan="2">

What EMOTION & BODY SENSATIONS do I feel/notice?

</td></tr>
<tr><td>

Where is this felt?

Size? Shape? Edges?

</td><td>

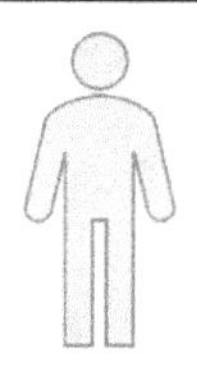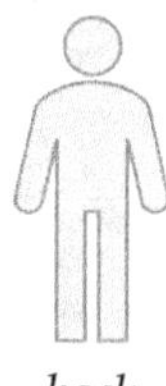

front   *back*

</td></tr>
<tr><td colspan="2">

Intensity of Emotion BEFORE tapping:

</td></tr>
<tr><td colspan="2">

1 2 3 4 5 6 7 8 9 10   Low – Medium – High

</td></tr>
</table>

SET UP STATEMENT: 3x's at side of hand

> "Even though
>
>
>
> ,*I deeply and completely accept myself"

Self-Acceptance Phrase

REMINDER PHRASE: at all other points

> "This   in my

CHECK INTENSITY OF EMOTION: check after each round

Set Up for Additional Tapping as needed

"Even though *I have some remaining* __________, I deeply and completely accept myself."

"This *remaining* _______.

NOTES: ______________________________________

____

____

____

____

____

____

____

____

Date___________

THE PROBLEM's "MOVIE TITLE"

THE NEGATIVE BELIEF/SELF-TALK:

Rate it: 1-100 (1= least intense, 100 = most intense)

CONSIDER THE DETAILS (past/present/future):

WHAT event/condition happened?   WHEN did it start?

WHO was/will be involved?   WHAT was/is going on?

WHERE did/will it happen?   WHY did/will it happen?

WHEN did/will it happen?   HOW did/will it happen?

What does this REMIND me of?   What OTHER ISSUES came up?

What is the EARLIEST MEMORY   What other SELF TALK attends
this reminds me of?   this?

What EMOTION & BODY SENSATIONS do I feel/notice?

Where is this felt?

Size? Shape? Edges?

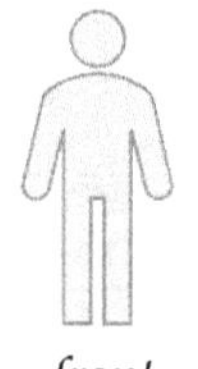 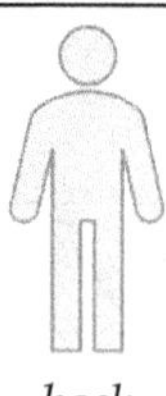

front   *back*

Intensity of Emotion BEFORE tapping:

1 2 3 4 5 6 7 8 9 10   Low – Medium – High

SET UP STATEMENT: 3x's at side of hand

"Even though

,*I deeply and completely accept myself"

Self-Acceptance Phrase

REMINDER PHRASE: at all other points

"This   in my

CHECK INTENSITY OF EMOTION: check after each round

Set Up for Additional Tapping as needed

"Even though *I have some remaining* __________, I deeply and completely accept myself."

"This *remaining* ________.

NOTES: ____

____

____

____

____

____

____

____

____

Date___________

THE PROBLEM's "MOVIE TITLE"

THE NEGATIVE BELIEF/SELF-TALK:

Rate it: 1-100 (1= least intense, 100 = most intense)

CONSIDER THE DETAILS (past/present/future):

WHAT event/condition happened?	WHEN did it start?
WHO was/will be involved?	WHAT was/is going on?
WHERE did/will it happen?	WHY did/will it happen?
WHEN did/will it happen?	HOW did/will it happen?

What does this REMIND me of?	What OTHER ISSUES came up?
What is the EARLIEST MEMORY this reminds me of?	What other SELF TALK attends this?

What EMOTION & BODY SENSATIONS do I feel/notice?

Where is this felt?

Size? Shape? Edges?

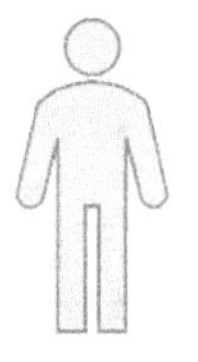 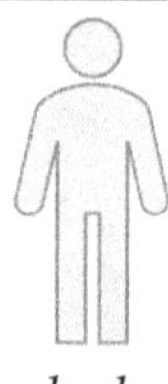

front   *back*

Intensity of Emotion BEFORE tapping:

1 2 3 4 5 6 7 8 9 10   Low – Medium – High

SET UP STATEMENT: 3x's at side of hand

"Even though

,*I deeply and completely accept myself"

Self-Acceptance Phrase

REMINDER PHRASE: at all other points

"This   in my

CHECK INTENSITY OF EMOTION: check after each round

Set Up for Additional Tapping as needed

"Even though *I have some remaining* _________, I deeply and completely accept myself."

"This *remaining* _______.

NOTES: ______________________________________

____

____

____

____

____

____

____

Date___________

<table>
<tr><td>

THE PROBLEM's "MOVIE TITLE"

</td></tr>
</table>

<table>
<tr><td>

THE NEGATIVE BELIEF/SELF-TALK:

</td></tr>
<tr><td>

Rate it: 1-100 (1= least intense, 100 = most intense)

</td></tr>
</table>

<table>
<tr><td colspan="2">

CONSIDER THE DETAILS (past/present/future):

</td></tr>
<tr><td>

WHAT event/condition happened?

WHO was/will be involved?

WHERE did/will it happen?

WHEN did/will it happen?

</td><td>

WHEN did it start?

WHAT was/is going on?

WHY did/will it happen?

HOW did/will it happen?

</td></tr>
<tr><td>

What does this REMIND me of?

What is the EARLIEST MEMORY this reminds me of?

</td><td>

What OTHER ISSUES came up?

What other SELF TALK attends this?

</td></tr>
</table>

<table>
<tr><td colspan="2">

What EMOTION & BODY SENSATIONS do I feel/notice?

</td></tr>
<tr><td>

Where is this felt?

Size? Shape? Edges?

</td><td>

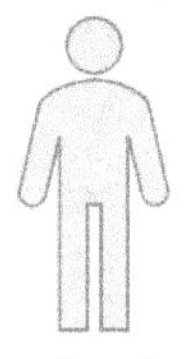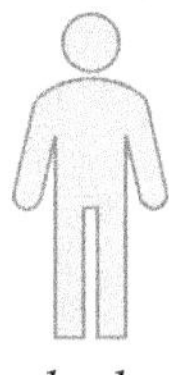

front   *back*

</td></tr>
<tr><td colspan="2">

Intensity of Emotion BEFORE tapping:

</td></tr>
<tr><td colspan="2">

1 2 3 4 5 6 7 8 9 10   Low – Medium – High

</td></tr>
</table>

SET UP STATEMENT: 3x's at side of hand

"Even though

,*I deeply and completely accept myself"

*Self-Acceptance Phrase

REMINDER PHRASE: at all other points

"This   in my

CHECK INTENSITY OF EMOTION: check after each round

Set Up for Additional Tapping as needed

"Even though *I have some remaining* __________, I deeply and completely accept myself."

"This *remaining* _______.

NOTES:

____

____

____

____

____

____

____

____

Date___________

THE PROBLEM's "MOVIE TITLE"

THE NEGATIVE BELIEF/SELF-TALK:

Rate it: 1-100 (1= least intense, 100 = most intense)

CONSIDER THE DETAILS (past/present/future):

WHAT event/condition happened?	WHEN did it start?
WHO was/will be involved?	WHAT was/is going on?
WHERE did/will it happen?	WHY did/will it happen?
WHEN did/will it happen?	HOW did/will it happen?

What does this REMIND me of?	What OTHER ISSUES came up?
What is the EARLIEST MEMORY this reminds me of?	What other SELF TALK attends this?

What EMOTION & BODY SENSATIONS do I feel/notice?

Where is this felt?

Size? Shape? Edges?

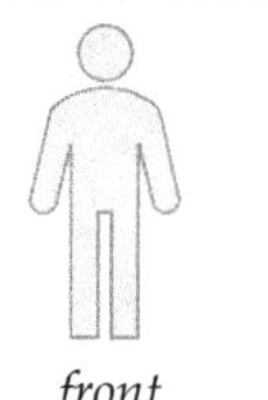
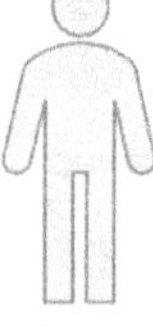

front   *back*

Intensity of Emotion BEFORE tapping:

1 2 3 4 5 6 7 8 9 10   Low – Medium – High

SET UP STATEMENT: 3x's at side of hand

"Even though

,*I deeply and completely accept myself"

Self-Acceptance Phrase

REMINDER PHRASE: at all other points

"This   in my

CHECK INTENSITY OF EMOTION: check after each round

Set Up for Additional Tapping as needed

"Even though *I have some remaining* __________, I deeply and completely accept myself."

"This *remaining* _______.

NOTES: ____

____

____

____

____

____

____

____

____

Date___________

THE PROBLEM's "MOVIE TITLE"

THE NEGATIVE BELIEF/SELF-TALK:

Rate it: 1-100 (1= least intense, 100 = most intense)

CONSIDER THE DETAILS (past/present/future):

WHAT event/condition happened?	WHEN did it start?
WHO was/will be involved?	WHAT was/is going on?
WHERE did/will it happen?	WHY did/will it happen?
WHEN did/will it happen?	HOW did/will it happen?

What does this REMIND me of?	What OTHER ISSUES came up?
What is the EARLIEST MEMORY this reminds me of?	What other SELF TALK attends this?

What EMOTION & BODY SENSATIONS do I feel/notice?

Where is this felt?

Size? Shape? Edges?

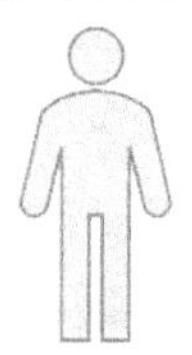 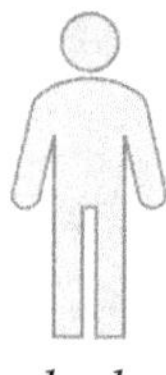

front   *back*

Intensity of Emotion BEFORE tapping:

1 2 3 4 5 6 7 8 9 10   Low – Medium – High

SET UP STATEMENT: 3x's at side of hand

"Even though

,*I deeply and completely accept myself"

Self-Acceptance Phrase

REMINDER PHRASE: at all other points

"This   in my

CHECK INTENSITY OF EMOTION: check after each round

Set Up for Additional Tapping as needed

"Even though ***I have some remaining*** ________, I deeply and completely accept myself."

"This ***remaining*** ______.

NOTES: ____

____

____

____

____

____

____

____

____

Date___________

THE PROBLEM's "MOVIE TITLE"

THE NEGATIVE BELIEF/SELF-TALK:

Rate it: 1-100 (1= least intense, 100 = most intense)

CONSIDER THE DETAILS (past/present/future):

WHAT event/condition happened?	WHEN did it start?
WHO was/will be involved?	WHAT was/is going on?
WHERE did/will it happen?	WHY did/will it happen?
WHEN did/will it happen?	HOW did/will it happen?

What does this REMIND me of?	What OTHER ISSUES came up?
What is the EARLIEST MEMORY this reminds me of?	What other SELF TALK attends this?

What EMOTION & BODY SENSATIONS do I feel/notice?

Where is this felt?

Size? Shape? Edges?

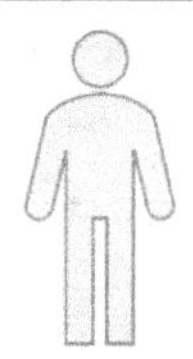 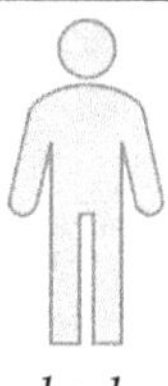

front   *back*

Intensity of Emotion BEFORE tapping:

1 2 3 4 5 6 7 8 9 10   Low – Medium – High

SET UP STATEMENT: 3x's at side of hand

"Even though

,*I deeply and completely accept myself"

Self-Acceptance Phrase

REMINDER PHRASE: at all other points

"This   in my

CHECK INTENSITY OF EMOTION: check after each round

Set Up for Additional Tapping as needed

"Even though *I have some remaining* __________, I deeply and completely accept myself."

"This *remaining* ________.

NOTES: ____

____

____

____

____

____

____

____

Date___________

THE PROBLEM's "MOVIE TITLE"

THE NEGATIVE BELIEF/SELF-TALK:

Rate it: 1-100 (1= least intense, 100 = most intense)

CONSIDER THE DETAILS (past/present/future):

WHAT event/condition happened?	WHEN did it start?
WHO was/will be involved?	WHAT was/is going on?
WHERE did/will it happen?	WHY did/will it happen?
WHEN did/will it happen?	HOW did/will it happen?

What does this REMIND me of?	What OTHER ISSUES came up?
What is the EARLIEST MEMORY this reminds me of?	What other SELF TALK attends this?

What EMOTION & BODY SENSATIONS do I feel/notice?

Where is this felt?
Size? Shape? Edges?

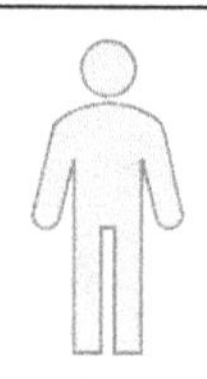 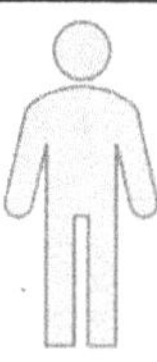

front   *back*

Intensity of Emotion BEFORE tapping:

1 2 3 4 5 6 7 8 9 10   Low – Medium – High

SET UP STATEMENT: 3x's at side of hand

"Even though

,*I deeply and completely accept myself"

Self-Acceptance Phrase

REMINDER PHRASE: at all other points

"This   in my

CHECK INTENSITY OF EMOTION: check after each round

Set Up for Additional Tapping as needed

"Even though *I have some remaining* _________, I deeply and completely accept myself."

"This *remaining* _______.

NOTES:

____

____

____

____

____

____

____

____

____

Date___________

THE PROBLEM's "MOVIE TITLE"

THE NEGATIVE BELIEF/SELF-TALK:

Rate it: 1-100 (1= least intense, 100 = most intense)

CONSIDER THE DETAILS (past/present/future):

WHAT event/condition happened?	WHEN did it start?
WHO was/will be involved?	WHAT was/is going on?
WHERE did/will it happen?	WHY did/will it happen?
WHEN did/will it happen?	HOW did/will it happen?

What does this REMIND me of?	What OTHER ISSUES came up?
What is the EARLIEST MEMORY this reminds me of?	What other SELF TALK attends this?

What EMOTION & BODY SENSATIONS do I feel/notice?

Where is this felt?

Size? Shape? Edges?

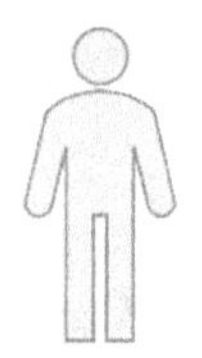

front

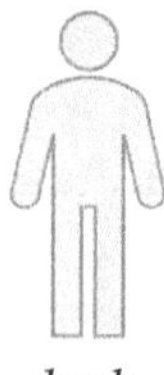

back

Intensity of Emotion BEFORE tapping:

1 2 3 4 5 6 7 8 9 10   Low – Medium – High

SET UP STATEMENT: 3x's at side of hand

> "Even though
>
>
>
>
>
>
> ,*I deeply and completely accept myself"

Self-Acceptance Phrase

REMINDER PHRASE: at all other points

"This   in my

CHECK INTENSITY OF EMOTION: check after each round

Set Up for Additional Tapping as needed

"Even though *I have some remaining* __________, I deeply and completely accept myself."

"This *remaining* ______.

NOTES: ______________________________________

____

____

____

____

____

____

____

____

Date______________

<table>
<tr><td>

THE PROBLEM's "MOVIE TITLE"

</td></tr>
</table>

<table>
<tr><td>

THE NEGATIVE BELIEF/SELF-TALK:

</td></tr>
<tr><td>

Rate it: 1-100 (1= least intense, 100 = most intense)

</td></tr>
</table>

<table>
<tr><td colspan="2">

CONSIDER THE DETAILS (past/present/future):

</td></tr>
<tr><td>

WHAT event/condition happened?

WHO was/will be involved?

WHERE did/will it happen?

WHEN did/will it happen?

</td><td>

WHEN did it start?

WHAT was/is going on?

WHY did/will it happen?

HOW did/will it happen?

</td></tr>
<tr><td>

What does this REMIND me of?

What is the EARLIEST MEMORY this reminds me of?

</td><td>

What OTHER ISSUES came up?

What other SELF TALK attends this?

</td></tr>
</table>

<table>
<tr><td colspan="2">

What EMOTION & BODY SENSATIONS do I feel/notice?

</td></tr>
<tr><td>

Where is this felt?
Size? Shape? Edges?

</td><td>

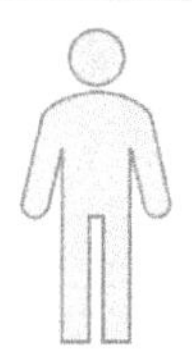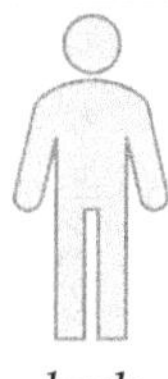

front   *back*

</td></tr>
<tr><td colspan="2">

Intensity of Emotion BEFORE tapping:

1 2 3 4 5 6 7 8 9 10   Low – Medium – High

</td></tr>
</table>

SET UP STATEMENT: 3x's at side of hand

"Even though

,*I deeply and completely accept myself"

Self-Acceptance Phrase

REMINDER PHRASE: at all other points

"This   in my

CHECK INTENSITY OF EMOTION: check after each round

Set Up for Additional Tapping as needed

"Even though *I have some remaining* __________, I deeply and completely accept myself."

"This *remaining* _______.

NOTES: ____

____

____

____

____

____

____

____

____

Date____________

THE PROBLEM's "MOVIE TITLE"

THE NEGATIVE BELIEF/SELF-TALK:

Rate it: 1-100 (1= least intense, 100 = most intense)

CONSIDER THE DETAILS (past/present/future):

WHAT event/condition happened?	WHEN did it start?
WHO was/will be involved?	WHAT was/is going on?
WHERE did/will it happen?	WHY did/will it happen?
WHEN did/will it happen?	HOW did/will it happen?

What does this REMIND me of?	What OTHER ISSUES came up?
What is the EARLIEST MEMORY this reminds me of?	What other SELF TALK attends this?

What EMOTION & BODY SENSATIONS do I feel/notice?

Where is this felt?

Size? Shape? Edges?

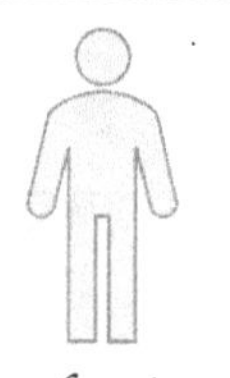 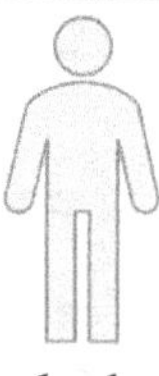

front   *back*

Intensity of Emotion BEFORE tapping:

1 2 3 4 5 6 7 8 9 10   Low – Medium – High

SET UP STATEMENT: 3x's at side of hand

"Even though

,*I deeply and completely accept myself"

*Self-Acceptance Phrase

REMINDER PHRASE: at all other points

"This   in my

CHECK INTENSITY OF EMOTION: check after each round

Set Up for Additional Tapping as needed

"Even though *I have some remaining* __________, I deeply and completely accept myself."

"This *remaining* ______.

NOTES: ____

____

____

____

____

____

____

____

____

Date___________

THE PROBLEM's "MOVIE TITLE"

THE NEGATIVE BELIEF/SELF-TALK:

Rate it: 1-100 (1= least intense, 100 = most intense)

CONSIDER THE DETAILS (past/present/future):

WHAT event/condition happened?	WHEN did it start?
WHO was/will be involved?	WHAT was/is going on?
WHERE did/will it happen?	WHY did/will it happen?
WHEN did/will it happen?	HOW did/will it happen?

What does this REMIND me of?	What OTHER ISSUES came up?
What is the EARLIEST MEMORY this reminds me of?	What other SELF TALK attends this?

What EMOTION & BODY SENSATIONS do I feel/notice?

Where is this felt?

Size? Shape? Edges?

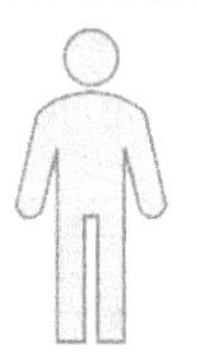
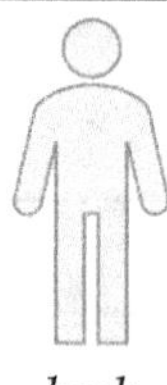

front   *back*

Intensity of Emotion BEFORE tapping:

1 2 3 4 5 6 7 8 9 10   Low – Medium – High

SET UP STATEMENT: 3x's at side of hand

"Even though

,*I deeply and completely accept myself"

*Self-Acceptance Phrase

REMINDER PHRASE: at all other points

"This   in my

CHECK INTENSITY OF EMOTION: check after each round

Set Up for Additional Tapping as needed

"Even though *I have some remaining* __________, I deeply and completely accept myself."

"This *remaining* _______.

NOTES: ____

____

____

____

____

____

____

____

____

Date___________

<table>
<tr><td>

THE PROBLEM's "MOVIE TITLE"

</td></tr>
</table>

<table>
<tr><td>

THE NEGATIVE BELIEF/SELF-TALK:

</td></tr>
<tr><td>

Rate it: 1-100 (1= least intense, 100 = most intense)

</td></tr>
</table>

<table>
<tr><td colspan="2">

CONSIDER THE DETAILS (past/present/future):

</td></tr>
<tr><td>

WHAT event/condition happened?

WHO was/will be involved?

WHERE did/will it happen?

WHEN did/will it happen?

</td><td>

WHEN did it start?

WHAT was/is going on?

WHY did/will it happen?

HOW did/will it happen?

</td></tr>
<tr><td>

What does this REMIND me of?

What is the EARLIEST MEMORY this reminds me of?

</td><td>

What OTHER ISSUES came up?

What other SELF TALK attends this?

</td></tr>
</table>

<table>
<tr><td colspan="2">

What EMOTION & BODY SENSATIONS do I feel/notice?

</td></tr>
<tr><td>

Where is this felt?

Size? Shape? Edges?

</td><td>

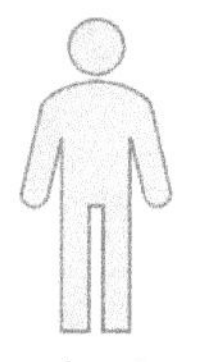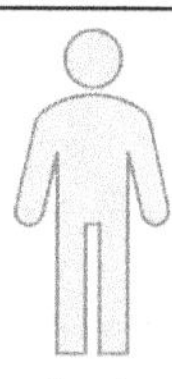

front   *back*

</td></tr>
<tr><td colspan="2">

Intensity of Emotion BEFORE tapping:

</td></tr>
<tr><td colspan="2">

1 2 3 4 5 6 7 8 9 10   Low – Medium – High

</td></tr>
</table>

SET UP STATEMENT: 3x's at side of hand

"Even though

,*I deeply and completely accept myself"

*Self-Acceptance Phrase

REMINDER PHRASE: at all other points

"This   in my

CHECK INTENSITY OF EMOTION: check after each round

Set Up for Additional Tapping as needed

"Even though *I have some remaining* __________, I deeply and completely accept myself."

"This *remaining* _______.

NOTES: ____________________________________

____

____

____

____

____

____

____

Date___________

THE PROBLEM's "MOVIE TITLE"

THE NEGATIVE BELIEF/SELF-TALK:

Rate it: 1-100 (1= least intense, 100 = most intense)

CONSIDER THE DETAILS (past/present/future):

WHAT event/condition happened?	WHEN did it start?
WHO was/will be involved?	WHAT was/is going on?
WHERE did/will it happen?	WHY did/will it happen?
WHEN did/will it happen?	HOW did/will it happen?

What does this REMIND me of?	What OTHER ISSUES came up?
What is the EARLIEST MEMORY this reminds me of?	What other SELF TALK attends this?

What EMOTION & BODY SENSATIONS do I feel/notice?

Where is this felt?

Size? Shape? Edges?

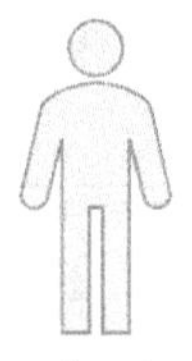
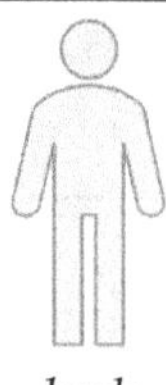

front   *back*

Intensity of Emotion BEFORE tapping:

1 2 3 4 5 6 7 8 9 10   Low – Medium – High

SET UP STATEMENT: 3x's at side of hand

"Even though

,*I deeply and completely accept myself"

Self-Acceptance Phrase

REMINDER PHRASE: at all other points

"This   in my

CHECK INTENSITY OF EMOTION: check after each round

Set Up for Additional Tapping as needed

"Even though *I have some remaining* _________, I deeply and completely accept myself."

"This *remaining* _______.

NOTES:

Date___________

THE PROBLEM's "MOVIE TITLE"

THE NEGATIVE BELIEF/SELF-TALK:

Rate it: 1-100 (1= least intense, 100 = most intense)

CONSIDER THE DETAILS (past/present/future):

WHAT event/condition happened?	WHEN did it start?
WHO was/will be involved?	WHAT was/is going on?
WHERE did/will it happen?	WHY did/will it happen?
WHEN did/will it happen?	HOW did/will it happen?

What does this REMIND me of?	What OTHER ISSUES came up?
What is the EARLIEST MEMORY this reminds me of?	What other SELF TALK attends this?

What EMOTION & BODY SENSATIONS do I feel/notice?

Where is this felt?

Size? Shape? Edges?

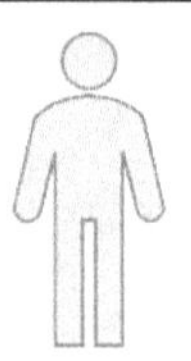
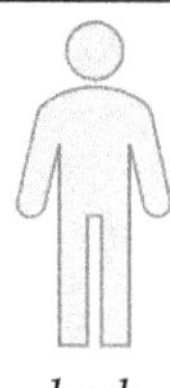

front　　*back*

Intensity of Emotion BEFORE tapping:

1 2 3 4 5 6 7 8 9 10　　　　Low – Medium – High

SET UP STATEMENT: 3x's at side of hand

"Even though

,*I deeply and completely accept myself"

Self-Acceptance Phrase

REMINDER PHRASE: at all other points

"This   in my

CHECK INTENSITY OF EMOTION: check after each round

Set Up for Additional Tapping as needed

"Even though *I have some remaining* _________, I deeply and completely accept myself."

"This *remaining* _______.

NOTES: ____

____

____

____

____

____

____

____

Date___________

THE PROBLEM's "MOVIE TITLE"

THE NEGATIVE BELIEF/SELF-TALK:

Rate it: 1-100 (1= least intense, 100 = most intense)

CONSIDER THE DETAILS (past/present/future):

WHAT event/condition happened?	WHEN did it start?
WHO was/will be involved?	WHAT was/is going on?
WHERE did/will it happen?	WHY did/will it happen?
WHEN did/will it happen?	HOW did/will it happen?

What does this REMIND me of?	What OTHER ISSUES came up?
What is the EARLIEST MEMORY this reminds me of?	What other SELF TALK attends this?

What EMOTION & BODY SENSATIONS do I feel/notice?

Where is this felt?

Size? Shape? Edges?

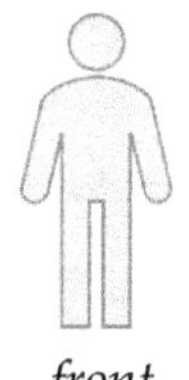 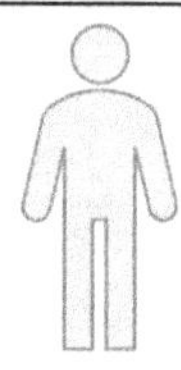

front   *back*

Intensity of Emotion BEFORE tapping:

1 2 3 4 5 6 7 8 9 10   Low – Medium – High

SET UP STATEMENT: 3x's at side of hand

"Even though

,*I deeply and completely accept myself"

Self-Acceptance Phrase

REMINDER PHRASE: at all other points

"This   in my

CHECK INTENSITY OF EMOTION: check after each round

Set Up for Additional Tapping as needed

"Even though *I have some remaining* __________, I deeply and completely accept myself."

"This *remaining* _______.

NOTES: ____

____

____

____

____

____

____

____

____

Date____________

<table>
<tr><td>

THE PROBLEM's "MOVIE TITLE"

</td></tr>
</table>

<table>
<tr><td>

THE NEGATIVE BELIEF/SELF-TALK:

Rate it: 1-100 (1= least intense, 100 = most intense)

</td></tr>
</table>

CONSIDER THE DETAILS (past/present/future):

WHAT event/condition happened?	WHEN did it start?
WHO was/will be involved?	WHAT was/is going on?
WHERE did/will it happen?	WHY did/will it happen?
WHEN did/will it happen?	HOW did/will it happen?

What does this REMIND me of?	What OTHER ISSUES came up?
What is the EARLIEST MEMORY this reminds me of?	What other SELF TALK attends this?

What EMOTION & BODY SENSATIONS do I feel/notice?

Where is this felt?

Size? Shape? Edges?

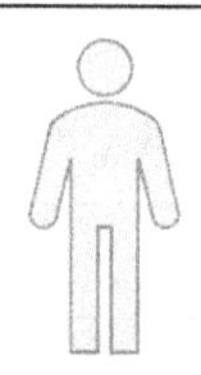 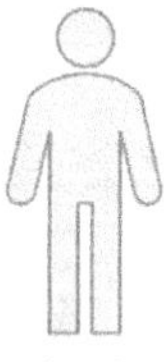

front   *back*

Intensity of Emotion BEFORE tapping:

1 2 3 4 5 6 7 8 9 10   Low – Medium – High

SET UP STATEMENT: 3x's at side of hand

> "Even though
>
>
>
>
>   ,*I deeply and completely accept myself"

Self-Acceptance Phrase

REMINDER PHRASE: at all other points

> "This   in my

CHECK INTENSITY OF EMOTION: check after each round

Set Up for Additional Tapping as needed

"Even though *I have some remaining* __________, I deeply and completely accept myself."

"This *remaining* _______.

NOTES: ____

____

____

____

____

____

____

____

Date___________

THE PROBLEM's "MOVIE TITLE"

THE NEGATIVE BELIEF/SELF-TALK:

Rate it: 1-100 (1= least intense, 100 = most intense)

CONSIDER THE DETAILS (past/present/future):

WHAT event/condition happened?	WHEN did it start?
WHO was/will be involved?	WHAT was/is going on?
WHERE did/will it happen?	WHY did/will it happen?
WHEN did/will it happen?	HOW did/will it happen?

What does this REMIND me of?	What OTHER ISSUES came up?
What is the EARLIEST MEMORY this reminds me of?	What other SELF TALK attends this?

What EMOTION & BODY SENSATIONS do I feel/notice?

Where is this felt?

Size? Shape? Edges?

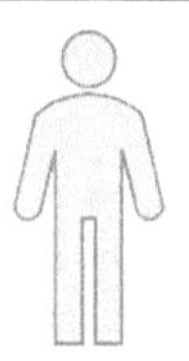
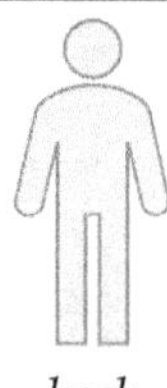

front   *back*

Intensity of Emotion BEFORE tapping:

1 2 3 4 5 6 7 8 9 10   Low – Medium – High

SET UP STATEMENT: 3x's at side of hand

> "Even though
>
>
>
>
> ,*I deeply and completely accept myself"

Self-Acceptance Phrase

REMINDER PHRASE: at all other points

> "This   in my

CHECK INTENSITY OF EMOTION: check after each round

Set Up for Additional Tapping as needed

"Even though *I have some remaining* __________, I deeply and completely accept myself."

"This *remaining* ________.

NOTES: ____

____

____

____

____

____

____

____

____

____

Date___________

THE PROBLEM's "MOVIE TITLE"

THE NEGATIVE BELIEF/SELF-TALK:

Rate it: 1-100 (1= least intense, 100 = most intense)

CONSIDER THE DETAILS (past/present/future):

WHAT event/condition happened?	WHEN did it start?
WHO was/will be involved?	WHAT was/is going on?
WHERE did/will it happen?	WHY did/will it happen?
WHEN did/will it happen?	HOW did/will it happen?

What does this REMIND me of?	What OTHER ISSUES came up?
What is the EARLIEST MEMORY this reminds me of?	What other SELF TALK attends this?

What EMOTION & BODY SENSATIONS do I feel/notice?

Where is this felt?
Size? Shape? Edges?

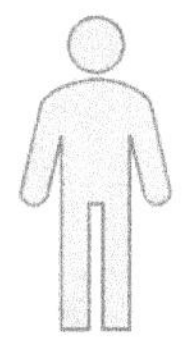 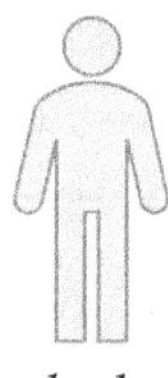

front   *back*

Intensity of Emotion BEFORE tapping:

1 2 3 4 5 6 7 8 9 10   Low – Medium – High

SET UP STATEMENT: 3x's at side of hand

"Even though

,*I deeply and completely accept myself"

Self-Acceptance Phrase

REMINDER PHRASE: at all other points

"This   in my

CHECK INTENSITY OF EMOTION: check after each round

Set Up for Additional Tapping as needed

"Even though *I have some remaining* __________, I deeply and completely accept myself."

"This *remaining* _______.

NOTES: ____

____

____

____

____

____

____

____

____

Date___________

THE PROBLEM's "MOVIE TITLE"

THE NEGATIVE BELIEF/SELF-TALK:

Rate it: 1-100 (1= least intense, 100 = most intense)

CONSIDER THE DETAILS (past/present/future):

WHAT event/condition happened?	WHEN did it start?
WHO was/will be involved?	WHAT was/is going on?
WHERE did/will it happen?	WHY did/will it happen?
WHEN did/will it happen?	HOW did/will it happen?

What does this REMIND me of?	What OTHER ISSUES came up?
What is the EARLIEST MEMORY this reminds me of?	What other SELF TALK attends this?

What EMOTION & BODY SENSATIONS do I feel/notice?

Where is this felt?

Size? Shape? Edges?

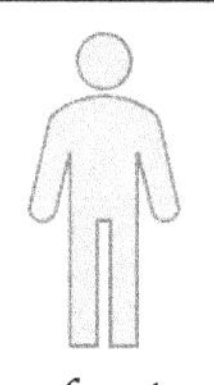 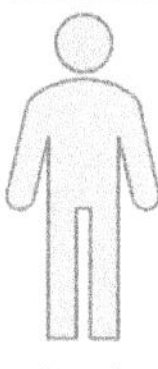

front   *back*

Intensity of Emotion BEFORE tapping:

1 2 3 4 5 6 7 8 9 10   Low – Medium – High

SET UP STATEMENT: 3x's at side of hand

> "Even though
>
>
>
>
>
> ,*I deeply and completely accept myself"

Self-Acceptance Phrase

REMINDER PHRASE: at all other points

> "This   in my

CHECK INTENSITY OF EMOTION: check after each round

Set Up for Additional Tapping as needed

"Even though *I have some remaining* ________, I deeply and completely accept myself."

"This *remaining* ______.

NOTES: ____

____

____

____

____

____

____

____

____

____

Date___________

<table>
<tr><td>

THE PROBLEM's "MOVIE TITLE"

</td></tr>
</table>

<table>
<tr><td>

THE NEGATIVE BELIEF/SELF-TALK:

</td></tr>
<tr><td>

Rate it: 1-100 (1= least intense, 100 = most intense)

</td></tr>
</table>

<table>
<tr><td colspan="2">

CONSIDER THE DETAILS (past/present/future):

</td></tr>
<tr><td>

WHAT event/condition happened?

WHO was/will be involved?

WHERE did/will it happen?

WHEN did/will it happen?

</td><td>

WHEN did it start?

WHAT was/is going on?

WHY did/will it happen?

HOW did/will it happen?

</td></tr>
<tr><td>

What does this REMIND me of?

What is the EARLIEST MEMORY this reminds me of?

</td><td>

What OTHER ISSUES came up?

What other SELF TALK attends this?

</td></tr>
</table>

<table>
<tr><td colspan="2">

What EMOTION & BODY SENSATIONS do I feel/notice?

</td></tr>
<tr><td>

Where is this felt?

Size? Shape? Edges?

</td><td>

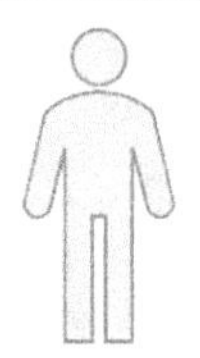 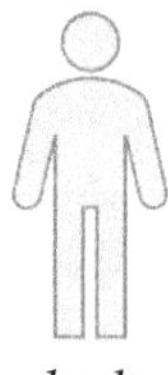

front   *back*

</td></tr>
<tr><td colspan="2">

Intensity of Emotion BEFORE tapping:

</td></tr>
<tr><td colspan="2">

1 2 3 4 5 6 7 8 9 10   Low – Medium – High

</td></tr>
</table>

SET UP STATEMENT: 3x's at side of hand

> "Even though
>
>
>
>
>
> ,*I deeply and completely accept myself"

Self-Acceptance Phrase

REMINDER PHRASE: at all other points

> "This   in my

CHECK INTENSITY OF EMOTION: check after each round

Set Up for Additional Tapping as needed

"Even though *I have some remaining* __________, I deeply and completely accept myself."

"This *remaining* ________.

NOTES: ____

____

____

____

____

____

____

____

____

____

Date___________

THE PROBLEM's "MOVIE TITLE"

THE NEGATIVE BELIEF/SELF-TALK:

Rate it: 1-100 (1= least intense, 100 = most intense)

CONSIDER THE DETAILS (past/present/future):

WHAT event/condition happened?	WHEN did it start?
WHO was/will be involved?	WHAT was/is going on?
WHERE did/will it happen?	WHY did/will it happen?
WHEN did/will it happen?	HOW did/will it happen?

What does this REMIND me of?	What OTHER ISSUES came up?
What is the EARLIEST MEMORY this reminds me of?	What other SELF TALK attends this?

What EMOTION & BODY SENSATIONS do I feel/notice?

Where is this felt?
Size? Shape? Edges?

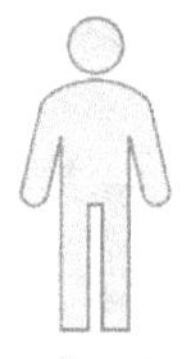 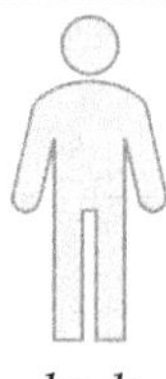

front   *back*

Intensity of Emotion BEFORE tapping:

1 2 3 4 5 6 7 8 9 10   Low – Medium – High

SET UP STATEMENT: 3x's at side of hand

"Even though

,*I deeply and completely accept myself"

Self-Acceptance Phrase

REMINDER PHRASE: at all other points

"This   in my

CHECK INTENSITY OF EMOTION: check after each round

Set Up for Additional Tapping as needed

"Even though ***I have some remaining*** ________, I deeply and completely accept myself."

"This ***remaining*** ______.

NOTES: ______________________________________

____

____

____

____

____

____

____

Date______________

THE PROBLEM's "MOVIE TITLE"

THE NEGATIVE BELIEF/SELF-TALK:

Rate it: 1-100 (1= least intense, 100 = most intense)

CONSIDER THE DETAILS (past/present/future):

WHAT event/condition happened?	WHEN did it start?
WHO was/will be involved?	WHAT was/is going on?
WHERE did/will it happen?	WHY did/will it happen?
WHEN did/will it happen?	HOW did/will it happen?

What does this REMIND me of?	What OTHER ISSUES came up?
What is the EARLIEST MEMORY this reminds me of?	What other SELF TALK attends this?

What EMOTION & BODY SENSATIONS do I feel/notice?

Where is this felt?

Size? Shape? Edges?

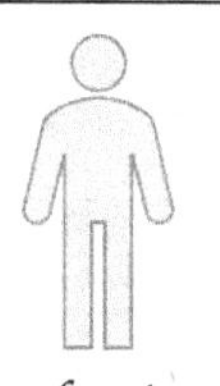 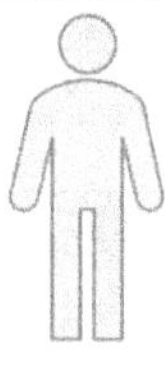

front   *back*

Intensity of Emotion BEFORE tapping:

1 2 3 4 5 6 7 8 9 10   Low – Medium – High

SET UP STATEMENT: 3x's at side of hand

> "Even though
>
>
>
>
>
> ,*I deeply and completely accept myself"

Self-Acceptance Phrase

REMINDER PHRASE: at all other points

> "This   in my

CHECK INTENSITY OF EMOTION: check after each round

Set Up for Additional Tapping as needed

"Even though *I have some remaining* _________, I deeply and completely accept myself."

"This *remaining* _______.

NOTES:

____

____

____

____

____

____

____

____

Date____________

THE PROBLEM's "MOVIE TITLE"

THE NEGATIVE BELIEF/SELF-TALK:

Rate it: 1-100 (1= least intense, 100 = most intense)

CONSIDER THE DETAILS (past/present/future):

WHAT event/condition happened?	WHEN did it start?
WHO was/will be involved?	WHAT was/is going on?
WHERE did/will it happen?	WHY did/will it happen?
WHEN did/will it happen?	HOW did/will it happen?

What does this REMIND me of?	What OTHER ISSUES came up?
What is the EARLIEST MEMORY this reminds me of?	What other SELF TALK attends this?

What EMOTION & BODY SENSATIONS do I feel/notice?

Where is this felt?

Size? Shape? Edges?

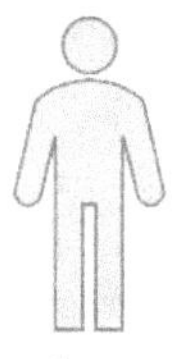 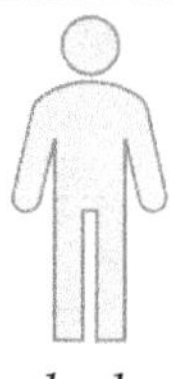

front   *back*

Intensity of Emotion BEFORE tapping:

1 2 3 4 5 6 7 8 9 10   Low – Medium – High

SET UP STATEMENT: 3x's at side of hand

"Even though

,*I deeply and completely accept myself"

Self-Acceptance Phrase

REMINDER PHRASE: at all other points

"This   in my

CHECK INTENSITY OF EMOTION: check after each round

Set Up for Additional Tapping as needed

"Even though *I have some remaining* __________, I deeply and completely accept myself."

"This *remaining* _______.

NOTES: ____

____

____

____

____

____

____

____

Date___________

THE PROBLEM's "MOVIE TITLE"

THE NEGATIVE BELIEF/SELF-TALK:

Rate it: 1-100 (1= least intense, 100 = most intense)

CONSIDER THE DETAILS (past/present/future):

WHAT event/condition happened?	WHEN did it start?
WHO was/will be involved?	WHAT was/is going on?
WHERE did/will it happen?	WHY did/will it happen?
WHEN did/will it happen?	HOW did/will it happen?

What does this REMIND me of?	What OTHER ISSUES came up?
What is the EARLIEST MEMORY this reminds me of?	What other SELF TALK attends this?

What EMOTION & BODY SENSATIONS do I feel/notice?

Where is this felt?
Size? Shape? Edges?

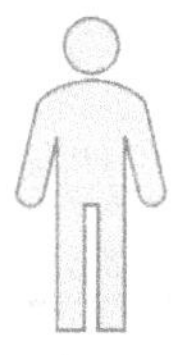
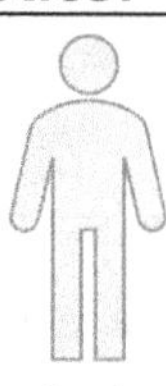

front   *back*

Intensity of Emotion BEFORE tapping:

1 2 3 4 5 6 7 8 9 10   Low – Medium – High

SET UP STATEMENT: 3x's at side of hand

"Even though

,*I deeply and completely accept myself"

Self-Acceptance Phrase

REMINDER PHRASE: at all other points

"This   in my

CHECK INTENSITY OF EMOTION: check after each round

Set Up for Additional Tapping as needed

"Even though *I have some remaining* __________, I deeply and completely accept myself."

"This *remaining* ______.

NOTES: ______________________________________

____

____

____

____

____

____

____

Date___________

THE PROBLEM's "MOVIE TITLE"

THE NEGATIVE BELIEF/SELF-TALK:

Rate it: 1-100 (1= least intense, 100 = most intense)

CONSIDER THE DETAILS (past/present/future):

WHAT event/condition happened?	WHEN did it start?
WHO was/will be involved?	WHAT was/is going on?
WHERE did/will it happen?	WHY did/will it happen?
WHEN did/will it happen?	HOW did/will it happen?

What does this REMIND me of?	What OTHER ISSUES came up?
What is the EARLIEST MEMORY this reminds me of?	What other SELF TALK attends this?

What EMOTION & BODY SENSATIONS do I feel/notice?

Where is this felt?

Size? Shape? Edges?

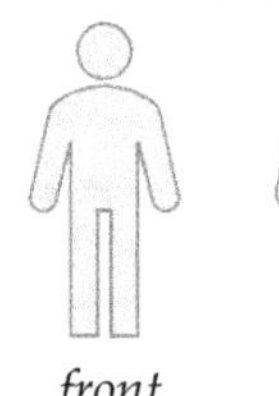 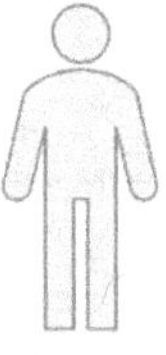

front   *back*

Intensity of Emotion BEFORE tapping:

1 2 3 4 5 6 7 8 9 10   Low – Medium – High

SET UP STATEMENT: 3x's at side of hand

> "Even though
>
>
>
>
> ,*I deeply and completely accept myself"

Self-Acceptance Phrase

REMINDER PHRASE: at all other points

> "This   in my

CHECK INTENSITY OF EMOTION: check after each round

Set Up for Additional Tapping as needed

"Even though *I have some remaining* _________, I deeply and completely accept myself."

"This *remaining* _______.

NOTES: _______________________________________

____

____

____

____

____

____

____

____

Date______________

THE PROBLEM's "MOVIE TITLE"

THE NEGATIVE BELIEF/SELF-TALK:

Rate it: 1-100 (1= least intense, 100 = most intense)

CONSIDER THE DETAILS (past/present/future):

WHAT event/condition happened?	WHEN did it start?
WHO was/will be involved?	WHAT was/is going on?
WHERE did/will it happen?	WHY did/will it happen?
WHEN did/will it happen?	HOW did/will it happen?

What does this REMIND me of?	What OTHER ISSUES came up?
What is the EARLIEST MEMORY this reminds me of?	What other SELF TALK attends this?

What EMOTION & BODY SENSATIONS do I feel/notice?

Where is this felt?

Size? Shape? Edges?

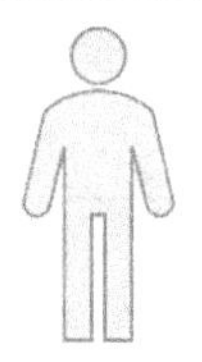
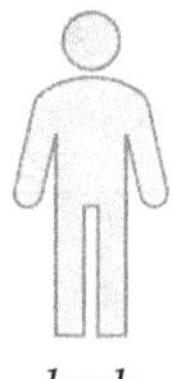

front   *back*

Intensity of Emotion BEFORE tapping:

1 2 3 4 5 6 7 8 9 10   Low – Medium – High

SET UP STATEMENT: 3x's at side of hand

"Even though

,*I deeply and completely accept myself"

Self-Acceptance Phrase

REMINDER PHRASE: at all other points

"This   in my

CHECK INTENSITY OF EMOTION: check after each round

Set Up for Additional Tapping as needed

"Even though *I have some remaining* ________, I deeply and completely accept myself."

"This *remaining* ______.

NOTES: ____

____

____

____

____

____

____

____

Date___________

<table>
<tr><td>

THE PROBLEM's "MOVIE TITLE"

</td></tr>
</table>

<table>
<tr><td>

THE NEGATIVE BELIEF/SELF-TALK:

</td></tr>
<tr><td>

Rate it: 1-100 (1= least intense, 100 = most intense)

</td></tr>
</table>

<table>
<tr><td colspan="2">

CONSIDER THE DETAILS (past/present/future):

</td></tr>
<tr><td>

WHAT event/condition happened?

WHO was/will be involved?

WHERE did/will it happen?

WHEN did/will it happen?

</td><td>

WHEN did it start?

WHAT was/is going on?

WHY did/will it happen?

HOW did/will it happen?

</td></tr>
<tr><td>

What does this REMIND me of?

What is the EARLIEST MEMORY this reminds me of?

</td><td>

What OTHER ISSUES came up?

What other SELF TALK attends this?

</td></tr>
</table>

<table>
<tr><td colspan="2">

What EMOTION & BODY SENSATIONS do I feel/notice?

</td></tr>
<tr><td>

Where is this felt?

Size? Shape? Edges?

</td><td>

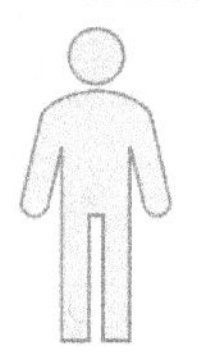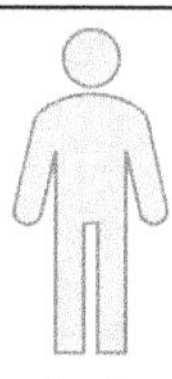

front   *back*

</td></tr>
<tr><td colspan="2">

Intensity of Emotion BEFORE tapping:

</td></tr>
<tr><td colspan="2">

1 2 3 4 5 6 7 8 9 10   Low – Medium – High

</td></tr>
</table>

SET UP STATEMENT: 3x's at side of hand

"Even though

,*I deeply and completely accept myself"

Self-Acceptance Phrase

REMINDER PHRASE: at all other points

"This   in my

CHECK INTENSITY OF EMOTION: check after each round

Set Up for Additional Tapping as needed

"Even though *I have some remaining* __________, I deeply and completely accept myself."

"This *remaining* _______.

NOTES: ______________________________________

____

____

____

____

____

____

____

____

NOTES, REFLECTIONS, INSIGHTS

~ Tap IT Out ~

ABOUT SHERLYNNE PUBLISHING

257

Hi, I'm SherLynne.

SherLynne Publishing (formerly Success Families) is where my book creations land. Typically, they're books I create to use in my own home. Since I find them useful, I think you might to, so I design these with you in mind as well.

The books are inspired by my drive to do better, one baby-step at a time. I believe that is accomplished through addressing mindset, stuck places in our mind and practice.

Some of my books come from making Christmas gifts (joke books) pretty journals, homeschool books for handwriting and copy-work, and other subjects, teaching mindset as I mentor individuals, and my own healing journey.

Feel free to follow along and stay in touch through my website: ***www.sherlynne.com***.

If there are specific journals, diaries, workbooks, or classes you'd like to have available, drop me a note. I'm always open to new ideas on how to serve my followers and their families!